# Walking The Weight Off

## FOR

## DUMMIES®

A Wiley Brand

by Erin Palinski-Wade

FOR

DUMMIES®
A Wiley Brand

**Walking The Weight Off For Dummies**®

Published by: **John Wiley & Sons, Inc.,** 111 River Street, Hoboken, NJ 07030-5774, www.wiley.com

Copyright © 2015 by John Wiley & Sons, Inc., Hoboken, New Jersey

Published simultaneously in Canada

No part of this publication may be reproduced, stored in a retrieval system or transmitted in any form or by any means, electronic, mechanical, photocopying, recording, scanning or otherwise, except as permitted under Sections 107 or 108 of the 1976 United States Copyright Act, without the prior written permission of the Publisher. Requests to the Publisher for permission should be addressed to the Permissions Department, John Wiley & Sons, Inc., 111 River Street, Hoboken, NJ 07030, (201) 748-6011, fax (201) 748-6008, or online at http://www.wiley.com/go/permissions.

**Trademarks:** Wiley, For Dummies, the Dummies Man logo, Dummies.com, Making Everything Easier, and related trade dress are trademarks or registered trademarks of John Wiley & Sons, Inc., and may not be used without written permission. All other trademarks are the property of their respective owners. John Wiley & Sons, Inc., is not associated with any product or vendor mentioned in this book.

LIMIT OF LIABILITY/DISCLAIMER OF WARRANTY: THE PUBLISHER AND THE AUTHOR MAKE NO REPRESENTATIONS OR WARRANTIES WITH RESPECT TO THE ACCURACY OR COMPLETENESS OF THE CONTENTS OF THIS WORK AND SPECIFICALLY DISCLAIM ALL WARRANTIES, INCLUDING WITHOUT LIMITATION WARRANTIES OF FITNESS FOR A PARTICULAR PURPOSE. NO WARRANTY MAY BE CREATED OR EXTENDED BY SALES OR PROMOTIONAL MATERIALS. THE ADVICE AND STRATEGIES CONTAINED HEREIN MAY NOT BE SUITABLE FOR EVERY SITUATION. THIS WORK IS SOLD WITH THE UNDERSTANDING THAT THE PUBLISHER IS NOT ENGAGED IN RENDERING LEGAL, ACCOUNTING, OR OTHER PROFESSIONAL SERVICES. IF PROFESSIONAL ASSISTANCE IS REQUIRED, THE SERVICES OF A COMPETENT PROFESSIONAL PERSON SHOULD BE SOUGHT. NEITHER THE PUBLISHER NOR THE AUTHOR SHALL BE LIABLE FOR DAMAGES ARISING HEREFROM. THE FACT THAT AN ORGANIZATION OR WEBSITE IS REFERRED TO IN THIS WORK AS A CITATION AND/OR A POTENTIAL SOURCE OF FURTHER INFORMATION DOES NOT MEAN THAT THE AUTHOR OR THE PUBLISHER ENDORSES THE INFORMATION THE ORGANIZATION OR WEBSITE MAY PROVIDE OR RECOMMENDATIONS IT MAY MAKE. FURTHER, READERS SHOULD BE AWARE THAT INTERNET WEBSITES LISTED IN THIS WORK MAY HAVE CHANGED OR DISAPPEARED BETWEEN WHEN THIS WORK WAS WRITTEN AND WHEN IT IS READ. SOME OF THE EXERCISES AND DIETARY SUGGESTIONS CONTAINED IN THIS WORK MAY NOT BE APPROPRIATE FOR ALL INDIVIDUALS, AND READERS SHOULD CONSULT WITH A PHYSICIAN BEFORE COMMENCING ANY EXERCISE OR DIETARY PROGRAM.

For general information on our other products and services, please contact our Customer Care Department within the U.S. at 877-762-2974, outside the U.S. at 317-572-3993, or fax 317-572-4002. For technical support, please visit www.wiley.com/techsupport.

Wiley publishes in a variety of print and electronic formats and by print-on-demand. Some material included with standard print versions of this book may not be included in e-books or in print-on-demand. If this book refers to media such as a CD or DVD that is not included in the version you purchased, you may download this material at http://booksupport.wiley.com. For more information about Wiley products, visit www.wiley.com.

Library of Congress Control Number: 2014958561

ISBN 978-1-119-00250-5 (pbk); ISBN 978-1-119-00254-3 (ebk); ISBN 978-1-119-00256-7 (ebk)

Manufactured in the United States of America

10  9  8  7  6  5  4  3  2  1

# Contents at a Glance

# Table of Contents

# Introduction

So you've decided you want to lose weight, right? And most likely, you've considered or tried various quick-fix weight-loss plans in the past only to lose weight and regain it shortly thereafter. If you're fed up with the weight-loss yo-yo game and are serious about losing weight and keeping it off, you need to focus on making healthy lifestyle changes you can stick with long term. And that's where this book comes in.

As a nutrition and fitness professional, I have worked with thousands of clients in the same situation as you. They may have had success with weight-loss plans but been unable to maintain the results. And one of the main reasons is that they were looking for a quick fix. Quick fixes just don't work. What does work is burning more calories than you take in. You see, weight loss doesn't have to be complicated — it's simple math. The key is to burn more calories so you don't have to drastically (or unrealistically) cut back on calories to a level that you can't maintain.

One of the easiest ways to burn more calories day in and day out is by walking. And the best part about it is that walking is one of the easiest, more versatile, and affordable forms of exercise you could ever ask for. That's why it's America's number-one form of exercise. It's easy to do anytime, any-where, and it works! Walking on a regular basis — whether going for a brisk, structured walk or just fitting in more steps every day — can help you shed pounds and inches and, most importantly, keep them off. That's why I wanted to write this book — to show you just how simple weight loss (and maintaining a healthy weight) really can be. And it all starts with just one easy step!

## About This Book

It probably comes as no surprise to you that exercise can help you lose weight. However, you may be unsure of just how much exercise or what type of exercise you need to lose weight. If you're new to exercise, you may also be unsure of how to get started. *Walking The Weight Off For Dummies* was designed specifically to answer these questions. Regardless of whether you're a seasoned exerciser looking to take your workout to the next level or have never exercised before, this book has something to offer you.

Unlike many weight-loss and fitness books on the market that provide strict, rigid guidelines that don't work for everyone, this book is completely customized to your needs. Using this book, you can begin to understand your exercise personality and goals and follow a personalized walking plan that not only will bring about quick results, but most importantly, will provide you with results you can maintain. When it comes to weight loss and exercise, the solution is not one-size-fits-all. This book addresses that fact, so no matter where you're starting from or how big or small your weight-loss goals are, you can achieve them once and for all.

This book is broken down into three main sections to help you lose weight: understanding how and why exercise promotes weight loss, determining the best exercise plan for your personal needs, and continuing to challenge yourself to maintain your results long term. You won't get to your goal weight with this book and wonder what's next. Instead, you'll find strategies and plans to help you not only get to your goal, but also to stay there for life. All of these sections work together to help you understand and achieve your weight-loss goals. However, each part, and even each chapter within each part, is entirely independent of the other chapters while providing you with helpful information. If you feel you're already knowledgeable in one area, feel free to skip it and dive right into the sections where you want to find out more. The great thing about this book is that there's no *right* place to start. You can start anywhere. Although a lot can be learned from starting at Chapter 1 and reading the book in order, you don't have to approach the book in this way. You can choose to read one chapter today, such as the one detailing individual walking plans, and then choose to read more about why walking is so effective at promoting weight loss another day.

As you read through this book, you'll notice that I flag some content as Technical Stuff and provide other information in the form of sidebars. This information can enhance your knowledge, but it's not critical for your weight-loss success. Skipping these areas is perfectly fine if you don't have the time to focus on them, and by doing so you won't miss any critical information.

Within this book, you may note that some web addresses break across two lines of text. If you're reading this book in print and want to visit one of these websites, simply key in the web address exactly as it's noted in the text, pretending as though the line break doesn't exist. If you're reading this as an e-book, you've got it easy — just click the web address to be taken directly to the website.

# Foolish Assumptions

I wrote this book with the assumption that you are looking to lose weight and improve your overall health. Because you were motivated enough to pick up this book, I assume that you've committed to making some lifestyle changes, even if only small ones, to start on the road to a healthier you. I also assume that, like everyone who wants to lose weight, you want to see results quickly. However, with that being said, I also assume you don't want to just see results quickly, but would like to maintain the results you achieve long term.

I never assume that you are foolish! In fact, I assume quite the opposite. You probably are already knowledgeable to some degree about weight loss and exercise, but would like guidance in these areas. I assume that you are most likely new to exercising as a form of weight loss or are already exercising some but looking for a way to enhance your results. I also assume that you have already made, or are considering making, improvements to your diet to help foster additional weight loss. However, if you're not sure how to eat to enhance your weight loss or have tried to make dietary changes unsuccessfully in the past, I encourage you to pick up my book *Belly Fat Diet For Dummies* along with the *Flat Belly Cookbook For Dummies* for individualized weight-loss plans that not only help to maximize your results when combined with the walking workouts in this book, but also further increase your knowledge of the role diet plays in weight loss and maintenance.

# Icons Used in This Book

In the margins of *Walking Off the Weight For Dummies* (as in all *For Dummies* books), you find icons to help you maneuver through the text. Here's what the icons mean.

Whether you're getting started with exercise, sticking with your walking plan, or working on maximizing your results, you'll find that I periodically point out tips and tricks to make achieving your results — and keeping them — as simple as possible.

Be careful! This icon calls your attention to health conditions that may make certain forms of exercise unsafe as well as points out ways to reduce your risk of injury while walking.

Here, I point out many of the "whys" concerning weight loss and health improvements, such as why walking is so effective. Although I find this information valuable, if you want, you can skip over this stuff and still not miss a beat.

When it comes to weight loss and improving health, at times you may find yourself feeling discouraged or sidetracked. You may also sometimes forget why you are working so hard to achieve your goals. The information highlighted here helps you remember what you are working so hard for and how to stay motivated throughout the process.

# Beyond the Book

This book provides a solid foundation for getting started with walking for weight loss. To maximize your results and stay motivated to continue with your walking plan, you may also want to check out additional resources available to you online:

- ✔ You can download the book's Cheat Sheet at www.dummies.com/cheatsheet/walkingtheweightoff. It's a handy resource to keep on your computer, tablet, or smartphone.

- ✔ You can read interesting companion articles that supplement the book's content at www.dummies.com/extras/walkingtheweightoff. I even include an extra top-ten list.

I also encourage you to check out my personal website, www.erinpalinski-author.com, for additional information, up-to-date research, product recommendations to enhance your walk, and weight-loss tips and recipes.

# Where to Go from Here

As with all *For Dummies* books, you can start at the first page of Chapter 1 or dive in anywhere the subject header grabs your attention. From there, you can move forward or backward as you like, skipping around or proceeding in sequence, to get everything you need from what's in store here.

If you don't plan to read in sequence from cover to cover, the obvious way to get your feet wet is to select the part that covers the subject you feel you need to explore most urgently and dive right in. Then dig into other sections that discuss subjects you feel you know pretty well, and you'll very likely discover some new facts or helpful tidbits. If you're really not sure what you hope to get from this book but know you want to begin working toward your weight-loss goals, start the old-fashioned way: Chapter 1 gives bite-sized overviews of just about everything else in the book, providing you with jumping-off points that help direct you where to go next.

# Part I
# Getting Started with Walking

# In this part . . .

- ✔ Find out just why walking is America's number one form of exercise.

- ✔ Discover the amazing health benefits of walking.

- ✔ Get the scoop on how walking can help you to shed pounds, lose inches, and most importantly, keep the weight off for good.

- ✔ Learn the various ways to incorporate walking into your daily routine.

# Chapter 1

# The Perfect Exercise: Walking

*O*ver 100 million people can't be wrong! Walking continues to be the number one form of exercise in America with over 100 million Americans walking regularly to improve fitness and manage their weight. Why is walking so popular? Is it the right exercise for you? As something that comes naturally to most of us, walking is a skill you already have. No need to take lessons, hire a trainer, or purchase expensive equipment. You already have everything you need to walk because you do it every day.

Walking is also a "no excuse" form of fitness. It can be done anywhere — around your home, at the grocery store, outside, at work, and so on. You can't say you couldn't exercise because you weren't able to get to the gym or forgot your exercise equipment. You can squeeze in a walk almost anytime no matter where you are. Talking on the phone? Stand and walk while you talk! Have to go grocery shopping? Take a few extra laps around the store before you get started. It's really that easy!

It sounds so simple to fit in a few minutes of walking here and there, but you may be wondering whether that can really make a difference. Does adding a few extra laps around the grocery store or walking while talking on the phone help you to shed pounds? The answer is "absolutely"!

Short walks, long walks, or just boosting daily movement by increasing your daily steps can do everything from help you shed pounds and unwanted inches to improve your overall health and even boost your mood and energy. Walking offers benefits to everyone at every age. That's the wonderful thing about walking. Whether you are a seasoned exerciser in great shape or just getting started with exercise, you can still reap weight loss and health benefits from walking. Throughout this book I help you identify just how walking can benefit you, and I give you tips and tricks to maximize your walking workout for the fastest results. You won't believe just how easy walking off the weight can really be!

# Why Walking?

You see it everywhere — on the nightly news, in articles in your local paper, or even just walking down the street. The obesity epidemic is on the rise. People of every age, including young children and teens, are affected. And one of the main reasons for this upward trend in obesity is the increase in sedentary lifestyles. Many people wake up in the morning, sit in their car or in a bus on their way to work, spend long hours at a desk job, and then commute home. After a long, stressful day, they may relax on the couch, watch TV, and then fall asleep.

Although the day may be busy, very little, if any, physical actitivity takes place. However, eating habits most likely remain unchanged. This imbalance of taking in more calories than you are burning due to inactivity leads to weight gain. Furthermore, it can have a dramatic impact on health as well.

So much, in fact, that one study found a sedentary lifestyle is now a bigger killer than cigarette smoking in our society!

As you can see, you owe it to yourself and your health to be more active. But with busy work schedules, family commitments, and day-to-day activities, how can you possibly make time to schedule in something else like regular exercise? That's where walking comes in! Walking is the number one exercise in our country for good reasons — it's easy to do, and you can do it anywhere, anytime! Right around your first birthday, you figured out how to put one foot in front of the other and walk around. Over the years, you've become an expert at walking. That's one reason it's such a great form of exercise — you already have all the skills you need to walk. Your body knows how to walk and your muscles are conditioned to walk; all you need to do is get up and walk more! Throughout this book, I show just why walking is the best exercise you can do, how you can do it anywhere at any time, and how it can have a major impact on your overall health as well as your body weight and waistline.

If you can walk anywhere, anytime, is any type of walking really exercise? For instance, if you are leisurely window shopping, is this just as much exercise as taking a brisk walk around the block? Or does hiking in the woods offer the best benefit to your health and body?

The answer is, when it comes to the definition of walking for exercise and fitness, all walking counts. This isn't to say that a casual stroll burns as many calories as a brisk uphill walk, but walking in any form contributes to your overall daily activity level and therefore your fitness level and health as well.

## Walking for daily living and fitness walking

When it comes to walking, there are many different forms. You can take a slow, leisurely walk; you can power walk; you can walk on an incline; you can even hike up a mountain. All of these are forms of walking that boost your overall daily calorie burn and health. That's one of the greatest benefits of walking. It can be adjusted to any fitness level and any location.

### Fitness walking

Fitness walking is defined as "the aerobic sport of brisk, rhythmic, vigorous walking, intended to improve cardiovascular efficiency, strengthen the heart, control weight gain, and reduce stress" by the American Heritage *Stedman's Medical Dictionary*. This type of walking is usually done for a set duration or time or for a set distance. When participating in fitness walking, you're aiming to walk to improve your overall fitness level, speed, and health. Fitness walking is usually done at a brisk pace, one at which you find your heart rate elevated and carrying on a full conversation may be difficult. This type of walking helps to burn the most calories per minute, and therefore can promote more rapid losses of weight and body fat.

### Walking for daily living

Walking is defined as "to advance or travel on foot at a moderate speed or pace" or "to move about or travel on foot for exercise or pleasure" by the Random House Dictionary. This type of general walking is the stop and go walking we all do throughout the day. You may walk through the grocery store or walk around your house as you clean. At work you may walk from your desk to the break room, or to speak with a coworker. Although this type of walking isn't always done at a brisk pace or with the intention of increasing fitness, it still plays a large role in weight management and overall health.

The amount of general walking you do throughout the day can be measured in individual steps versus distance or length of time. Using steps to measure your total activity throughout the day can make increasing exercise more manageable. Stating that you will walk an extra 1,000 steps during the day can sound more doable than saying you will add an extra half mile walk.

In fact, working in extra steps during the day instead of trying to schedule additional exercise makes walking less of a chore and more just another part of your day. Adding those extra steps is something you're more likely to stick with, allowing it to have a greater impact on your health and your body weight.

Throughout this book, I show you just how much increasing your daily steps can add up when it comes to weight loss as well as improving health. In Chapter 2, I provide you with an in-depth look at how increasing your steps can torch excess calories and the best ways to track and increase these steps over time. You see why research has found that daily active living, such as taking the stairs over the elevator or parking farther away at the store, may have even greater health benefits than short, intensive workouts that are counterbalanced by a day generally filled with sitting.

## The importance of walking for good health

Walking is not America's number one form of exercise for no reason. In fact, walking offers tremendous benefits to your health, your waistline, and even your mood and stress levels. To be honest, you can't afford not to walk! Now, if you've picked up this book, I'm sure the main benefit you're concerned about with walking is shedding pounds and inches. Well, don't worry — walking will certainly help you with this.

As you may already be aware from past failed weight-loss attempts, it's almost impossible to lose weight and keep it off long term with diet alone. Exercise needs to be a vital part of your daily routine. The formula for weight loss is simple. Take in fewer calories than you burn and you'll lose weight. However, the more active you are, the more calories you burn, which allows more flexibility with your eating plan. You can cut calories without exercise and lose weight, but keeping this weight off without exercise can be quite challenging. Exercising on a regular basis helps to build and maintain muscle mass. Because muscle boosts metabolism (the amount of calories you burn each day), increasing it makes weight management easier.

To show you just how important physical activity is to weight loss, take a study done at Wake Forest University Medical Center. This study compared two groups of women: one group who dieted and one who walked while dieting. The women who walked between 1 and 2 miles daily three times per week were able to shrink stubborn belly fat cells by 18 percent over a four month period, while those who just dieted showed no change in belly fat cells. As you can see by these results, just short walks a few times per week can make a large difference in body fat as well as body weight.

In addition to weight loss, walking offers many other health benefits as well including:

- ✔ Improving heart health
- ✔ Lowering stress levels
- ✔ Decreasing diabetes risk
- ✔ Improving bone health
- ✔ Boosting mood
- ✔ Improving cognitive function
- ✔ Boosting the immune system
- ✔ Decreasing symptoms associated with menopause
- ✔ Improving sleep
- ✔ Increasing lifespan

# The Benefits of Walking as Exercise

If there were something you could do every day, something you already knew how to do, that was easy, didn't cost you a thing, could be done anywhere, and could help you shed pounds and improve health, would you do it? Who wouldn't? That's why walking is so popular! In just a few minutes per day, without buying any exercise equipment or having to travel to a gym, or learn a skill that requires the coordination of a circus acrobat, you can burn calories, shed inches, boost metabolism, and fight disease — just by putting one foot in front of the other! So why not get started today?

When you look at starting an exercise routine, the number one question you should ask yourself is "Is this something I can stick with?" With walking, the answer is usually an easy "yes."

Walking is a low-impact exercise, so even if you suffer from joint pain or have a history of injury, it's typically an exercise you can enjoy without risk of further injury or increased pain. Walking can also be as intense or as easy as you want. For instance, if one day you just don't feel like partaking in vigorous exercise, you can still boost your fitness level with a leisurely stroll around the park or the shopping mall. If you feel like an intense workout another day, you can power walk on an incline to really challenge your endurance.

As you can see, walking really offers something for everyone. It's an exercise you can do at any age or any fitness level. You can walk alone, in a group, or with a friend. Walking can take place outside in your neighborhood or a local park, indoors in a shopping center or around your home, at the gym on a treadmill, or even when traveling and sightseeing. Other than proper footwear, little equipment is required. With walking, there really are no excuses. Nothing is holding you back from fitting walking into your day. So are you ready to start moving?

## *You can walk anytime, almost anywhere*

Although taking the stairs instead of the elevator or walking the long way to the restroom at the office may not seem like exercise, it can all start to add up. That's one of the main reasons that walking is such a great form of exercise — it can really become part of your daily routine. In fact, once you get in the habit of increasing your daily physical activity by upping your daily steps, you'll be amazed at the results you can see from what feels like very little effort.

Unlike some forms of exercise where you have to schedule time, purchase equipment, or drive to the gym, walking can be done anywhere at any time. With walking, you move in a natural way that's fun and relaxing, without having to worry about learning special techniques or operating special equipment. And even if you've never exercised before, you know how to walk. In fact, I can almost guarantee you do it every day. So they only thing that is holding you back from increasing the amount you walk each day so you can start to drop pounds and inches is you.

Walking is such a popular form of exercise because it doesn't feel like "exercise" at all. In fact many experts now are starting to promote the idea of just getting more active to become fit than recommending we all "work out." One of the biggest reasons for this is compliance and consistency. If you think of the word "exercise" as something you dread doing or as a chore, motivating yourself to get started can be hard. Or, once you have started, it can be hard to stick with it if you aren't enjoying yourself. On the other hand, if you can simply take more steps today than you did the day before, that's easy! It doesn't feel like a chore. In fact, it seems almost too simple not to do. And that's what makes it so easy to stick with. Regardless of what you do to be more active, just being more physically active and staying that way will help you to lose weight, decrease belly fat, and improve your health and overall well-being.

## Almost anyone can do it

Even the most novice exerciser can take comfort in the fact that almost anyone can start a walking routine. The simplicity of walking is what makes it such a natural choice for exercise. It's a great way to gain confidence because it's beneficial to your health without being too challenging. And this is especially important if you are new to exercise or feel as though you're out of shape and want to ease back into exercise gradually.

With walking, you can make your workout whatever you want. If you want to focus on easing into exercise gradually, you can focus on building the amount of steps you take each day to increase your daily activity level. If you want to really challenge yourself, you can power walk to increase your speed, strength, and endurance. You can even change your terrain, such as by walking uphill or hiking through the woods, to add an extra level to your workout. One of the greatest things about walking is that it can be as easy or as challenging as you want it to be. And regardless of how you walk, the more you do it, the more benefits you'll gain.

Don't be fooled into thinking that if you don't go to the gym or get out and run for hours on end that you won't be able to shed pounds or get rid of stubborn belly fat. In fact, an hour at the gym may not even trump a day filled with many steps when it comes to weight loss. A study from the University of South Carolina found that women who spent about three quarters of their day being physically active (such as cleaning, running errands, and gardening) burned 10 percent more calories throughout the day than women who spent one hour at the gym but were sedentary the majority of the day otherwise. The research doesn't lie — walking really adds up! So no matter your age, your fitness level, or whether you are a gym rat or have never exercised a day in your life, just get up and put one foot in front of the other and start walking. It really is as easy as that!

# Deciding Whether Walking Is the Right Exercise for You

If you have opened this book, you are most likely considering walking as your primary source of exercise. If you're still contemplating whether walking is the right exercise for you, ask yourself the following questions:

- When you think about any form of exercise you can do, what do you consider the most enjoyable?
- What would be the easiest for you to fit into your daily routine?

✔ What exercise would be the least taxing on your body and your joints?

✔ What is an exercise you can do anywhere no matter whether you are at work, at home, or traveling?

If you think about all the many forms of exercise you can partake in, walking is one of the only ones that answers most, if not all, of these questions. Walking is easy. You already know how to do it. It can be done anywhere, anytime with no equipment needed. It's cheap, it's enjoyable, and you can do it alone or with others. Maybe instead of asking yourself whether walking is the right exercise for you, you may want to ask who walking is *not* a great choice of exercise for.

If you've been hesitant to get started with walking, ask yourself what may be holding you back. Is it the idea of trying to schedule yet another thing into your busy day? If so, walking doesn't need to be hard and you don't even need to "make time" for it per se. Walking can be as simple as tracking and increasing your steps by using a tool such as a pedometer. Check out Chapter 2 for more details on how to use a pedometer and how to work on increasing your daily steps to burn more calories without even realizing it!

If you've been resistant to start a walking routine for fear of getting off track due to having failed at past attempts to exercise, don't worry. Even if you were not successful with starting or sticking with an exercise routine in the past, it doesn't mean you can't be now.

One of the easiest ways to be successful with exercise is to make it a part of your daily routine and to make it as easy as possible. You can't get much easier than doing something you already do anyway. As with any exercise plan, you want to ease your way into a walking routine. You don't need to start walking for hours on end day after day (and that isn't even needed to see results). Instead, throughout this book I show you the best ways to get started and stick with your routine. You won't believe how easy it is to get moving and start seeing results!

## Assessing your exercise needs

When starting an exercise routine, you first want to assess your needs. What are you hoping to get out of your exercise plan? And more importantly, what does your exercise plan need to offer in order for you to stick with it? Walking can really be tailored to meet most of your exercise wants and needs. Once you identify what you want to get out of your walking routine, I can then help you identify the walking program that's best suited for you and your goals.

As you begin to think about what your walking routine needs to offer, ask yourself the following questions:

✔ Do I need an exercise I can do anywhere?

✔ Am I willing to use exercise equipment, or do I want to keep my workout as minimal as possible?

✔ Do I need to be only outdoors or only indoors when I exercise, or can my routine be flexible?

✔ Do I want my routine to help me tone and build muscle?

✔ Do I want my routine to improve my flexibility?

✔ Is my main desire for my routine to burn as many calories as possible in the shortest amount of time?

✔ Do I want an intense workout or a more relaxing workout?

✔ Is it important that my exercise routine incorporate a workout partner or buddy?

✔ Does my workout need to be as effective as possible in a very small time frame?

✔ Do I want to space my exercise out throughout the day or do it all at once?

✔ What is the most important factor in my workout routine to ensure I will be consistent with it?

Answering these questions can help you determine why you want to walk and what results are the most important for you to see from walking. Your answers to these questions will also help you to identify what type of walking routine will be the most enjoyable for you and the most likely for you to stick with. As with anything, consistency is key to achieving and maintaining results. For this reason, making sure you know just what type of walking routine you are most likely to be consistent with is key to your long-term success.

## Assessing your fitness level

Now that you know what you want your walking routine to offer you and the type of walking routine you will be most successful with, it's time to analyze your current fitness level. If you have never exercised in the past, you may be feeling slightly hesitant about starting. However, the beauty of walking is that it's a form of exercise you already do each and every day. No need to learn any fancy exercise techniques or be in a room full of fitness buffs where you feel intimidated. You can start at your own pace anywhere you want.

If you've never exercised before and have a mostly sedentary lifestyle, consider yourself a beginner when it comes to starting a walking routine. You can advance as quickly as you like; however, setting your expectations too high too soon can lead to burnout, causing you to fail to stick with your exercise routine.

If you're someone who doesn't regularly exercise but you have a very active life, such as working a physically active job, you may be able to start with a more challenging walking routine as your level of strength and endurance is higher than someone who is mainly sedentary.

If you already exercise by walking or another form of exercise, you can also jump into a more challenging walking routine. But regardless of your current fitness level, remember that when it comes to starting a new workout, don't try too much too soon.

Overexercising, especially in the beginning, can lead to injury, soreness, and a decreased likelihood of sticking to your workout routine. Start small and build up gradually, which is the best way to ensure you will be walking for years to come!

As you assess your current fitness level, it's important to consider any health conditions you may have, any past or current injuries, or any limitations such as joint pain that may impact your walking routine. As you read through this book, you find out what forms of walking for fitness are best for all fitness levels, health conditions, and even joint and bone conditions.

However, even if you have no prior health concerns, you should always contact your physician before starting or changing any exercise routine.

# Goal Setting and Walking

In order to be successful with an exercise routine, you need to understand why you are doing it. What motivated you to pick up this book? Have you always wanted to walk for exercise, but not known how? Are you trying to shed pounds and inches and thought this may work for you? Are you looking to improve your health or increase your energy levels? Whatever your reasons for exercising are, you want to identify them and remember them.

As you get started with your walking plan and continue with it over time, you want to look back at these reasons for exercise and see the progress you have made. For instance, if your main reason to start a walking routine is to lose inches around your waistline, in a month when your waistline is 2 inches smaller, you can use that result to motivate you to keep moving. If your goal is to lower your blood pressure and a few months from now you're able to decrease your medication dosage, you want to realize what a huge impact walking has had on your health so you can be motivated to continue with it.

When it comes to walking, you may have only one reason to get started or you may have many. What's most important is that you identify and remember these reasons. On a day when you're feeling sluggish and tired or just don't feel like walking, thinking about these reasons, the progress you have made, and the progress you still want to make, can help you stick with your routine. If, at times, you feel like you're working to increase your steps everyday and wonder whether it really makes a difference, you can look back at the pounds you've lost or how much lower your cholesterol level is and know that your efforts really have been paying off.

# Why goal setting is vital to walking success

You have made a commitment to yourself to start a walking routine. In order to not just start, but to also stick with this routine, you want to create a list of goals. When you compile your goal list, keep in mind that setting a goal isn't just about the end result. Small goals, even daily goals, are really what help you to achieve your long-term goals.

Take a look at an example: Mary wants to start walking to lose 40 pounds and decrease her blood pressure. Now, if every day, while Mary is lacing up her sneakers, all she thinks about is how much more weight she has to lose to reach her long-term goal of 40 pounds or how many more months it may be before she can get off her blood pressure medication, she may become discouraged. In fact, she may feel that her goals are so far off that they're not attainable and give up all together.

What can Mary do to get motivated and stay motivated with her walking routine so she can eventually reach her long-term goals? The answer is to set more goals! It may seem redundant, but setting small goals can help you achieve larger goals over time. In the journey to achieve your long-term goals, these small goals also help you feel a sense of accomplishment, which helps you stay on track and motivated. Mary may want to start by setting a goal of just walking, regardless of the time, daily. Just getting up and walking, even if only for a few minutes each day, means that she is on her way to being consistent with a walking routine. After she has achieved this goal, she can set a goal to walk for a minimum of 10 minutes per day. Before she knows it, she'll be down 5 pounds, and can focus on a goal of losing the next five. These small goals continuously give her something to work toward and achieve to keep her motivated. By using goal setting in this way, she is working toward her long-term goals every day but isn't becoming discouraged by the time it may take her to achieve them.

Goal setting can work in the same way for you and help to make you successful with your walking plan as well as your long-term goals. To set goals for yourself, start by asking yourself, "What was my main motivation for picking up this book?" Whatever the reason, take out a piece of paper and write it down. Now write down what you want to get out of exercise. Write down every benefit you are hoping for: weight loss, increased energy, improved health, a smaller waistline, fewer medications, and so on. As you write down your goals, make sure they are as specific as possible. If you want to lose weight, how much weight do you want to lose? If you want to decrease your cholesterol level, what is your cholesterol goal? If you are hoping your waistline will decrease, how many inches do you want to shed? Now, keep this list on hand because you'll use it as I show you just how walking can help you to achieve all of these goals.

## How walking can help you achieve your goals

After creating a list of all the goals you have for yourself, from weight loss to improved health and everything in between, it's time to focus on how walking can help you to achieve these goals. Walking can impact your body in a number of amazing ways. Walking can do all of the following and more:

- Increase the amount of calories you burn each day
- Tone muscles
- Boost metabolism
- Improve mood
- Decrease stress
- Lower blood pressure
- Decrease heart rate
- Lower blood sugar
- Improve overall cholesterol levels
- Decrease the risk of certain cancers
- Improve bone density
- Increase energy levels

The goals you set for yourself help to determine how you should walk, how often you should walk, what type of walking you should do, and even where you may want to walk. For instance, if you want to start a walking routine to stay at a healthy body weight and increase energy, your walking routine will look a bit different than that of the person who wants to build muscle and lose 20 pounds.

The more tailored your walking routine is to you and your goals, the quicker you'll see results and the more likely you are to maintain your results in the long run as well. And that's what I'm here to help you with. Throughout this book, I help you figure out the best walking plan for your fitness level and goals. Not only do I show you just how to get started and stick with this routine until you reach your goals, but I also show you how to maintain your results thereafter.

After you know what you want to get out of your walking routine and all the great things walking can do for you, it's time to break down your goals, look at each of them in depth, and determine just what style of walking will help you to achieve each goal.

Your goals for your walking routine most likely fall into one of three categories:

- ✔ Weight-loss goals
- ✔ Health goals
- ✔ Fitness goals

The type of goal you set impacts the walking routine you set for yourself. For instance, if you set a weight-loss goal of losing 10 pounds and a fitness goal of increasing your endurance, you want to make sure your walking routine not only focuses on burning more calories but is also challenging enough to improve your cardiovascular fitness to increase endurance. If someone else set a similar weight-loss goal but her only other goal was to decrease stress, her walking routine may focus more on increasing daily movement and long, leisurely walks.

Understanding what category the goals you set for yourself fall into is critical in determining how you design your walking routine. These goals also help you see how you should adjust your walking routine over time to help you reach all of your goals as quickly and easily as possible. It's also important to look at each goal you set for yourself and review it critically. Make sure the goals you set are realistic for you to achieve. Make sure those goals are healthy and safe. For instance, setting a goal to weigh well below your recommended ideal body weight is neither safe nor healthy. Setting a high-reaching goal such as walking 10 miles a day may be achievable, but is it really realistic to believe that you'll have time for this every day? Over time, walking this far day to day may also start to have a negative impact on your joints.

Be honest with yourself about what you can realistically achieve. Setting goals that are too lofty is doing a disservice to yourself by setting yourself up for failure. Start by setting realistic goals that challenge you, but are attainable. Remember, you can always add onto your goals at a later date.

### Your weight-loss goals

If you have picked up this book, most likely your main motivation for walking is to shed pounds and inches. Just how much weight you want to lose is up to you. However, when setting weight-loss goals, it's important to be realistic with yourself. You never want to aim for too low of a body weight, as that can be just as dangerous as being overweight. You also want to realize that the number on the scale is determined by many factors. Your age, height, bone structure, and even muscle mass all play a role in how much you weigh in addition to your level of body fat. A large-boned, muscular 5-foot, 6-inch person should never set a goal to weigh the same amount as a small-framed person of the same height. It just isn't realistic.

So what is a healthy weight range for you? If you focus solely on your weight on the scale, you may be missing the bigger picture. Someone who is of a normal weight can still have a large amount of body fat, in some instances more than another person who is slightly overweight. And vice versa: Someone who is "overweight" on a scale may have a large amount of muscle mass or a heavy bone structure, but a low percentage of body fat.

Although you don't want to disregard the scale entirely, you do want to be aware that it's not telling you the whole story. Other numbers are much more important for you to focus on when determining a weight-loss goal for yourself. One of these numbers is your BMI, or body mass index. It's a formula that takes into account your height versus your weight to determine whether you are at a healthy weight, underweight, or overweight. Although BMI can be a fairly reliable indicator of body fat in most people, there are exceptions. People with a very high level of muscle mass (mostly high-level athletes and bodybuilders) may have an elevated BMI without actually having a high level of body fat.

The easiest way to determine your BMI is to use the chart in Figure 1-1. The numbers on the left-hand side correlate with your height in inches. The numbers within the chart correlate with your body weight in pounds. To determine your BMI, find your height in inches, then scroll over until you reach your weight in pounds. Once you find where these intersect, draw your finger upward to the top of the chart to see what your BMI is. For instance, if you are 67 inches in height and weigh 189 pounds, your BMI is 29.

| BMI (kg/m²) | 19 | 20 | 21 | 22 | 23 | 24 | 25 | 26 | 27 | 28 | 29 | 30 | 35 | 40 |
|---|---|---|---|---|---|---|---|---|---|---|---|---|---|---|
| Height (in.) | Weight (lb.) | | | | | | | | | | | | | |
| 58 | 91 | 96 | 100 | 105 | 110 | 115 | 119 | 124 | 129 | 134 | 138 | 143 | 167 | 191 |
| 59 | 94 | 99 | 104 | 109 | 114 | 119 | 124 | 128 | 133 | 138 | 143 | 148 | 173 | 198 |
| 60 | 97 | 102 | 107 | 112 | 118 | 123 | 128 | 133 | 138 | 143 | 148 | 153 | 179 | 204 |
| 61 | 100 | 106 | 111 | 116 | 122 | 127 | 132 | 137 | 143 | 148 | 153 | 158 | 185 | 211 |
| 62 | 104 | 109 | 115 | 120 | 126 | 131 | 136 | 142 | 147 | 153 | 158 | 164 | 191 | 218 |
| 63 | 107 | 113 | 118 | 124 | 130 | 135 | 141 | 146 | 152 | 158 | 163 | 169 | 197 | 225 |
| 64 | 110 | 116 | 122 | 128 | 134 | 140 | 145 | 151 | 157 | 163 | 169 | 174 | 204 | 232 |
| 65 | 114 | 120 | 126 | 132 | 138 | 144 | 150 | 156 | 162 | 168 | 174 | 180 | 210 | 240 |
| 66 | 118 | 124 | 130 | 136 | 142 | 148 | 155 | 161 | 167 | 173 | 179 | 186 | 216 | 247 |
| 67 | 121 | 127 | 134 | 140 | 146 | 153 | 159 | 166 | 172 | 178 | 185 | 191 | 223 | 255 |
| 68 | 125 | 131 | 138 | 144 | 151 | 158 | 164 | 171 | 177 | 184 | 190 | 197 | 230 | 262 |
| 69 | 128 | 135 | 142 | 149 | 155 | 162 | 169 | 176 | 182 | 189 | 196 | 203 | 236 | 270 |
| 70 | 132 | 139 | 146 | 153 | 160 | 167 | 174 | 181 | 188 | 195 | 202 | 207 | 243 | 278 |
| 71 | 136 | 143 | 150 | 157 | 165 | 172 | 179 | 186 | 193 | 200 | 208 | 215 | 250 | 286 |
| 72 | 140 | 147 | 154 | 162 | 169 | 177 | 184 | 191 | 199 | 206 | 213 | 221 | 258 | 294 |
| 73 | 144 | 151 | 159 | 166 | 174 | 182 | 189 | 197 | 204 | 212 | 219 | 227 | 265 | 302 |
| 74 | 148 | 155 | 163 | 171 | 179 | 186 | 194 | 202 | 210 | 218 | 225 | 233 | 272 | 311 |
| 75 | 152 | 160 | 168 | 176 | 184 | 192 | 200 | 208 | 216 | 224 | 232 | 240 | 279 | 319 |
| 76 | 156 | 164 | 172 | 180 | 189 | 197 | 205 | 213 | 221 | 230 | 238 | 246 | 287 | 328 |

**Figure 1-1:**
Body mass
index chart.

© John Wiley & Sons, Inc.

Now that you know your BMI, what does this number mean? BMI has five categories. As you can see in the chart in Table 1-1, your BMI can fall into one of the following categories: underweight, healthy weight, overweight, obese, or morbidly obese. Your goal is to keep your BMI within the healthy weight range, because weighing too much or too little can increase your risk of many health complications.

| Table 1-1 | BMI Categories and Risk | |
|---|---|---|
| *BMI* | *Weight Status* | *Risk* |
| 18.5 or less | Underweight | Increased risk |
| 18.6–24.9 | Healthy weight | Low risk |
| 25.0–29.9 | Overweight | Increased risk |
| 30.0–39.9 | Obese | High risk |
| 40.0 or more | Morbid obesity | Very high risk |

Although BMI doesn't measure body fat directly, research has indicated that BMI does correspond with direct measures of body fat. If you have a high BMI but feel it may be elevated due to a high level of muscle mass, you can analyze your waist circumference to determine whether you have excess body fat or are at a healthy weight. Having a wide waistline indicates that you have excess visceral fat, otherwise known as belly fat. Too much of this fat has been associated with an increased risk for heart disease, type 2 diabetes, and even certain cancers. For these reasons, a healthy waist circumference is essential. The goals for waist circumference are as follows:

✔ **Men:** Under 40 inches

✔ **Women:** Under 35 inches

For individuals of Asian descent, the waist circumference goals are a little smaller:

✔ **Men:** Under 35 inches

✔ **Women:** Under 31 inches

To determine your waist circumference and see whether you may be at risk of having too much visceral fat, it's important to take an accurate measurement. To measure your waist, follow these steps:

**1. Locate your upper hipbone.**

**2. Place a tape measure around your bare stomach just above the upper hipbone (as shown in Figure 1-2).**

Make sure the measuring tape is parallel to the floor (slanting can falsely increase your measurement). Ensure that the tape measure is snug to your body, but not so tight it compresses the skin. Also make sure that you're exhaling and your abdomen is relaxed — no sucking in!

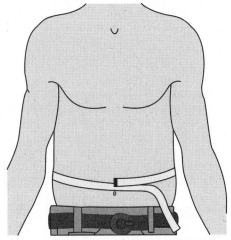

**Figure 1-2:** Measuring your waist circumference.

© John Wiley & Sons, Inc.

Once you determine your current BMI and waist circumference, you can use these numbers to help you create your weight-loss goals. If your BMI is greater than 30kg/m$^2$ (kilograms divided by meters squared), your first goal may be to reach a BMI of 29kg/m$^2$. If your waist circumference is 43 inches and you are female, you may want to make your first goal to decrease this measurement to 40 inches. Once you reach that goal, you can set a second goal to bring the measurement down under 35 inches. Setting realistic, attainable goals is much easier when you know what to aim for.

## Your health goals

Just as it can be hard to set a weight-loss goal without knowing what a healthy weight range is for you, the same can be said for setting health-related goals. You may know you want to lower your blood pressure or reduce cholesterol, but what cholesterol and blood pressure levels should you aim for? What about blood sugar? You may know an elevated blood sugar increases your risk for diabetes, but do you know what your level should be? Can too low be dangerous too?

The answer to the last question is yes. Just as having certain health measurements that are too high can increase disease risk, having readings that are too low can also have health implications. For instance, a blood-sugar range lower than normal can lead to feelings of shakiness, increased hunger, anxiousness, fainting, and in extreme cases, coma or death. When setting health goals for yourself, lower doesn't always mean better. You want to aim for an ideal range, and once you reach it, be able to stay in that range. Although certain health conditions, such as heart disease or diabetes, have specific health markers and lab work you can use to gauge your level of success, there are a few health measurements that almost everyone can use to determine disease risk and current state of health: cholesterol, blood pressure, and blood sugar (glucose).

### Cholesterol

Cholesterol is a waxy, fatlike substance produced by the liver and found in all the body's cells. It is also found in some of the foods you eat. Cholesterol is needed to make vitamin D as well as many hormones. In your body, substances called *lipoproteins* package and transport cholesterol to your cells.

Two kinds of lipoproteins that carry cholesterol in your body are high-density lipoproteins (HDL) and low-density lipoproteins (LDL). Having a healthy ratio of these lipoproteins is important to your health. HDL cholesterol, otherwise known as the "happy" cholesterol, is the cholesterol you want to have a high amount of. This form of cholesterol is like a garbage truck, picking up and transporting cholesterol back to the liver, which then removes cholesterol from your body. LDL cholesterol, or "lousy" cholesterol, is the one you want to have less of. High levels of this cholesterol can lead to a buildup of cholesterol in your arteries, which over time may lead to deadly blockages.

Knowing your cholesterol levels is important, as elevated levels may increase your risk of heart disease. In addition to knowing your levels of HDL and LDL cholesterol, you also want to assess two additional blood lipids: total cholesterol and triglycerides. *Total cholesterol* is a measurement of HDL cholesterol, LDL cholesterol, and other lipid components. *Triglycerides* are the fats flowing through your bloodstream from the food you eat. You should aim to have your levels of total cholesterol, LDL, HDL, and triglycerides checked annually or more often if elevated.

### Blood pressure

Blood pressure is just like its name: It's the measurement of the blood's force against the wall of the arteries. Two numbers make up blood pressure: systolic pressure and diastolic pressure. *Systolic pressure* is a measurement taken as the heart beats, whereas *diastolic pressure* is the measurement as the heart relaxes in between beats. The measurement is written as the systolic number over the diastolic number.

Elevated blood pressure (also known as *hypertension*), if not controlled, can increase risk for heart disease, stroke, and even kidney disease. It's important to have your blood pressure checked at least once annually and more often if elevated.

### Blood Sugar

Elevated blood sugar, also known as *glucose,* is a sign of insulin resistance, a precursor to type 2 diabetes. High amounts of glucose in the bloodstream can lead to serious health consequences including diabetes, heart disease, and kidney disease.

Having your blood glucose checked on a regular basis is key to preventing and controlling diabetes. If your blood glucose is found to be elevated, dietary changes, exercise, and decreasing belly fat have been shown to help reverse insulin resistance and lower blood glucose levels. Have glucose levels checked annually and more regularly if they are found to be elevated.

Using the ideal ranges for cholesterol, blood pressure, and blood glucose, you can create healthy and realistic health-related goals for yourself to work toward achieving. For more information on these health measures, see Chapter 18.

### Your fitness goals

When you start an exercise program, you may be tempted to set lofty goals. If you start walking and really enjoy it, you may want to aim for a 10K (kilometer) or even a half marathon. You may want to build strength, speed, and endurance. And all of these things will come. You will get stronger, build muscle, increase your speed and endurance, and even be able to tackle an event like a half marathon! But just like with anything, achieving these goals takes time. You can't expect to go from sitting on the couch one day to winning a 10K the next — no one can! But it doesn't mean you'll never be able to achieve completing a 10K. You certainly can if that's your desire, but it's all about taking small steps — literally!

Take a look at your long-term fitness goals. Then ask yourself how you will achieve them. How long do you realistically think it will take you to reach your goals? Say you feel as though you can achieve your fitness goals in three months, which is a reasonable time frame. Well, what is going to keep you motivated during that three-month period of time? It won't be thinking of your long-term goal every day. That would be more discouraging than anything! To keep you motivated, you need to develop small, achievable goals as you work toward the long-term goal. For example, say you want to walk faster. A plan to increase speed may look like the following:

1. **Start by walking for 15 minutes each day at a comfortable speed for one week.**

2. **After one week, track the distance you cover while walking for 15 minutes using a pedometer. Write down how many steps you cover while walking during this time frame (for example, 1,200 steps).**

3. **Aim to increase your speed to cover 100 additional steps in the 15 minute time frame over the course of the next week.**

   For example, from 1,200 steps you'd build up to 1,300 steps in 15 minutes.

4. **Continue to increase your speed by taking an additional 100 steps per walk each week until you can reach a goal of walking 2,000 steps in 15 minutes.**

   For instance, in Week 1 you walk 1,200 steps in 15 minutes, in Week 2 you walk 1,300 steps in 15 minutes, in Week 3 you walk 1,400 steps in 15 minutes, and so on until you achieve your goal.

You can use this same structure to achieve almost any fitness goal. For instance, maybe you want to increase the calorie burn of each walk by adding an incline. You can start walking on a flat surface, such as a treadmill, and raise the incline by 1 percent every week until you can walk at a 10 percent incline consistently. Or you can work on building your endurance by increasing the length of time you walk by extending your walk by 5 minutes each week. As you can see, these tiny goals add up to build results over time.

# Chapter 2

# The Health Benefits of Walking

## In This Chapter

▶ Understanding how walking can prevent disease

▶ Determining the impact walking has on mental health

▶ Discovering how walking can improve physical health

▶ Adapting your walking workout to your age

▶ Working walking into your lifestyle

*W*hat if there were something you could do — something you already do anyway — that, in just 30 minutes a day, could slash your risk for suffering a heart attack or stroke by as much as 30 to 40 percent and lower your risk of developing some cancers by as much as 30 percent? Would you do it? Could you afford not to? Would you be surprised to know that all you have to do to gain these amazing health benefits is walk?

There may never be a miracle pill that you can easily pop to drop pounds, shed inches, and fight disease, but there's always walking. Walking can offer all of these benefits and more, and it's so simple to do. You're already doing it anyway, so why not start making it work for you? Whether you're hoping to reduce body weight, shrink belly fat, fight disease, boost mood, or all of the above, walking will help you get there. All you have to do is make a commitment to walk regularly. It really is as easy as that!

Since humans' days as cavemen roaming the Earth, people have been up and walking. It's something your body does naturally. And, based on research study after research study, your body needs to keep walking in order to stay healthy and fight disease. Study after study has found that walking on a regular basis can do everything from fight heart disease to prevent diabetes, to even fight certain cancers and age-related cognitive decline. And physical health isn't the only thing that walking can impact. Walking has also been associated with a decreased risk of depression, can help you fight stress, and can even boost your mood. Every part of your body — from your heart to your brain, your muscles, and your bones — benefits from walking on a regular basis.

# Preventing Disease by Walking

Heart disease is the number one killer of both men and women in America. The Centers for Disease Control and Prevention (CDC) estimate more than one third (or 78.6 million) U.S. adults are obese. In addition, 26 million Americans have diabetes, and the American Cancer Society reports 1,638,910 new cancer cases and 577,190 deaths in 2012.

Many of these diseases are related to inactivity, poor diet, and weight gain and in fact, are the leading causes of preventable death in our country.

The key word here is *preventable*. These diseases don't have to be so prevalent. Eating well, maintaining a healthy weight, and of course being physically active can all help to prevent these diseases. And, if you have already been diagnosed, being physically active can help to control many of these diseases to improve both quality and quantity of life. One study published in the Archives of Internal Medicine found that walking just 30 minutes most days of the week can increase lifespan by up to three years. This section takes a look at just how much of an impact walking on a regular basis can have on preventing and treating these disease states.

## The impact on heart disease

The impact of heart disease on America is staggering. It's estimated that 935,000 Americans suffer a heart attack annually and the cost of coronary artery disease alone is over $108 billion dollars! So you can see just how widespread this problem really is. But there is a bright side: You can manage and even prevent heart disease simply by walking it away. In fact, just moderate amounts of walking daily can turn back your heart's clock. One study at Washington University found just that when it tracked people between the ages of 50 and 60 years old. They followed these individuals for one and a half years and found that those who walked enough to burn 240 to 300 calories per day had hearts that pumped nutrients and blood throughout the body as effectively as individuals in their 30s and 40s!

It's possible that walking may have a bigger role in improving heart health than even more intensive exercises such as jogging. For instance, one study comparing walkers to joggers who both exercised for the same amount of time and with the same frequency, found that walkers were able to lower triglyceride levels, the free fat within the bloodstream that, when elevated, can increase heart disease and diabetes risk, by twice as much! This may be due to a lower-intensity exercise, such as walking, burning more fat for fuel during exercise than higher-intensity exercises, such as running, which rely more on sugar (glucose) in the bloodstream for energy.

So how much walking does it take to improve your heart health? Surprisingly, not a lot. In just 30 minutes per day, one study found that walkers were able to significantly lower the inflammatory marker *C-reactive protein,* which is an independent marker for heart disease. As you can see, with just a small amount of effort and a little time, you can turn back your heart's clock and protect it against deadly heart disease all by just putting one foot in front of the other.

## Making a positive impact on diabetes

Inactivity is one of the leading causes of *insulin resistance,* which is a condition in which a person's body has a diminished response to the hormone insulin. This hormone is what the body uses to regulate *glucose* (sugar) in the body. When your body's cells become resistant to insulin, they don't allow it to carry glucose into your cells for energy. This resistance results in your body producing increased quantities of insulin as well as rising levels of glucose in the bloodstream.

Insulin resistance raises the risk of many diseases, including heart disease, diabetes, Alzheimer's disease, and even certain cancers. Between 60 and 70 million Americans have some level of insulin resistance, including one in every two adults over the age of 65, putting them well on their way to joining the 23.6 million Americans who already have diabetes. But just as with heart disease, insulin resistance and diabetes can be prevented and managed by simply walking.

Research has shown time and time again that walking can have a dramatic impact on your overall health. One study revealed that for those already suffering from insulin resistance, just getting up and moving by walking reduced the odds of developing type 2 diabetes by as much as 58 percent! Other research at the University of Michigan found that when sedentary adults started walking one hour per day, they were able to increase insulin sensitivity (the cells' ability to accept insulin) by as much as 59 percent. In addition, walking can help you reduce body weight and shed belly fat, both of which, when elevated, are risk factors for type 2 diabetes.

## Having an impact on cancer

A cancer diagnosis can be devastating for anyone. Although cancer can have a genetic component, many lifestyle factors can increase your risk for developing cancer.

Being overweight, being inactive, smoking, and eating a diet rich in red meat or low in fruits and vegetables can all increase your risk. However, many things you do every day can also help to prevent cancer. Leading a physically active lifestyle, regardless of your body weight, can have a protective effect in the fight against cancer.

Certain cancers seem to be impacted by walking more than others, one of which is breast cancer. The American Cancer Society found that by walking seven hours per week, you can lower your risk of developing breast cancer after menopause by 14 percent. Even more surprising is that this study found that even if women were overweight or gained weight during the study, the act of walking still decreased their cancer risk. Colon cancer and exercise also appear to have a significant link. Some research suggests that people who are physically active on a regular basis can decrease their risk of colon cancer by about 25 percent. These individuals are also less likely to develop polyps of the colon, which can become cancerous over time. Some evidence also points to physical activity decreasing the risk of prostate and lung cancer.

As compelling as the evidence is, you may be asking yourself why exercise, such as walking, makes such an impact on cancer risk. One reason, especially when it comes to colon cancer, is that increased physical activity helps to promote regular bowel movement which allows carcinogens in undigested food to pass through the bowel more quickly. As I mention earlier, exercise such as walking also lowers insulin resistance. When insulin is elevated in your body, it may encourage the growth of tumors. Therefore, decreasing the amount of insulin circulating in the body by decreasing insulin resistance may help to protect against cancer growth.

## Determining your risks

As you get started with an exercise routine and begin to walk on a regular basis, making sure you're healthy enough for physical activity is vital. In addition to consulting your healthcare professional for clearance to start or change an exercise routine, you may also want to assess your current health and establish a baseline. You can then measure changes in your health when you first start your walking routine, as you progress, and after you achieve your ultimate goals to see the improvements walking can make not only to your weight but also to your overall health.

When it comes to ordering lab tests to assess and monitor changes in your health, you can contact your physician, or you can now even order these tests on your own through many of the reputable websites that sell LapCorp tests.

## Additional health benefits

In addition to helping prevent diseases such as heart disease and diabetes, walking offers many other health benefits as well. One is its ability to help reduce and manage stress. Suffering from chronically elevated levels of stress over a long period of time can start to have a negative impact on your body and your health.

Elevated stress levels can increase blood pressure, lead to weight gain and increased belly fat, and even cause gastrointestinal symptoms such as constipation and diarrhea. Walking can help you to better manage stress and reduce the associated negative health consequences. Research has found that by walking, you can reduce anxiety and increase the levels of serotonin and dopamine in the body, which are basically "feel-good chemicals" in the brain. Elevating these brain chemicals can fight stress, decrease muscle tension, and decrease anxiety.

Walking can also help to impact sleep. Poor sleep or getting too little sleep has been associated with accelerated aging as well as an increased risk of weight gain. If you suffer from insomnia or are a generally poor sleeper, walking may be the key to a more restful night. One study in the Journal of Sleep Medicine shows just how powerful even a small amount of walking can be on sleep. It found that women age 60 and older woke up half as often and slept on average 48 minutes longer when walking just one hour per week as compared to women of the same age who were sedentary. In addition, other research has shown a decrease in nighttime waking and nightmares in individuals who walk on a regular basis. All of this increased quality of sleep results in a more rested you, who is healthier, happier, and better able to handle stress. In addition, direct links have been found between poor sleep and fatigue and food cravings and increased body weight. So it's quite possible that by improving the quality and quantity of your sleep you can actually rest away the pounds and inches!

For women who suffer from the symptoms of menopause such as hot flashes, weight gain, and night sweats, walking may offer some relief. One study found that performing moderate exercise, such as walking three hours per week, helped to reduce menopause-related symptoms. In addition, other research found that women who walked just 25 minutes per day suffered less menopause-related weight gain and headaches than those who walked less than 10 minutes per day.

As you can see, no matter your age, current weight, or lifestyle, walking offers benefits from cutting stress to fighting disease and everything in between. It doesn't take much, either — just a few minutes per day, and you'll be on your way to a healthier you!

# Sharpening and Soothing Your Mind

Your mind is an amazing thing! It can impact every aspect of your body from your mood to your energy levels, your stress levels, and even your physical well-being. You mind impacts your ability to think, to complete a task, to concentrate, and even your level of productivity during the day. The sharper your mind is, the easier it is for you to not only carry on your day-to-day activities easily and effectively, but to also remain in the best state of health. However, just like every other organ in your body, your brain needs you to take care of it so it can take care of you. The foods you eat, your stress levels, and your level of physical activity every day play a major role in how your brain functions.

If you are don't take care of your body properly, you may find that your mind is impacted. You may find that you're having a harder time processing your thoughts, or perhaps that you can't multitask as well as you once did. You may find your memory lapsing or find yourself experiencing a "cloudy" feeling when thinking. You may suffer from mood swings, such as feeling happy one minute and agitated the next. If any of these sound like you, you may be amazed to know that by simply walking, you can improve your mind, your mood, and even your memory! In this section, we show you how.

## *How walking can improve your mood*

Exercise can play a major role in your overall mood as it helps to boost *endorphins,* or "feel-good" chemicals in the brain. The term *runner's high* refers to this process too — a boost in these endorphins after exercise, which essentially provides you with a feeling of euphoria. Well, running isn't the only form of exercise that can make you feel good. Walking may actually help to lift mood more than running! Research found that walkers reported feeling better than their running counterparts not only after completing exercise, but while doing it as well. And this lift in mood isn't short-lived. Just 20 minutes of moderate intensity exercise, such as walking, has been found to be enough to provide your body with increased energy and a lifted mood for as much as 12 hours!

Walking may also help in the fight against depression. About 9 percent of American adults suffer from depression according to the CDC. In addition, about 3 percent of adults suffer from major depression, which is a long-lasting, severe form of depression and the leading cause of disability in Americans between the ages of 15 and 44 years.

Although medical intervention and treatment is often necessary to manage depression, walking may help in the fight against this disease as well.

One study found that by walking just 30 minutes per day, individuals with major depression reported a 40 percent improvement in well-being and an 85 percent increase in energy levels as opposed to those who did not walk. Walking for just 30 minutes per day five days per week has been found to boost energy, help adults feel more confident and healthier, and even improve their ability to complete daily tasks — all traits that can help to lift mood and fight depressive symptoms. In fact, exercise can play such a major role in the fight against depression that research has shown burning off just 350 calories three times per week though moderate exercise, such as walking, can reduce the symptoms of depression almost as effectively as antidepressant medication. Exercise such as walking can also work in combination with therapy and medications to control and treat severe depression.

Another benefit of walking on a regular basis, especially outdoors, is an increase in vitamin D levels. A deficiency of vitamin D has been linked with an increased risk of depression as well as seasonal affective disorder (SAD). Although vitamin D is available in some foods, such as dairy products, many people, especially those who work indoors or live in the northern hemisphere where sunlight is limited during parts of the year, are at risk of deficiency. Having your vitamin D levels tested and monitored can help you determine whether your levels are low and additional vitamin D supplementation or increased sun exposure may be needed. Discuss having your vitamin D levels checked with your physician or order a vitamin D test inexpensively and easily online. You can see a complete listing of labs that offer this service on my website at www.erinpalinski-author.com. Always discuss the results with your healthcare provider before adding or changing any supplement.

## How walking can sharpen your mind

Walking doesn't just lift your mood and spirits; it also helps to improve how your mind functions as well. Many studies have shown time and time again that moderate exercise, such as walking, can improve memory and concentration in everyone from young children to individuals in their 80s and beyond. No matter what your age or your current exercise level, adding walking to your daily routine can only help to sharpen your mind.

Short energy bursts of exercise lasting from 10 to 40 minutes have been shown to provide an immediate boost in mental focus and concentration. This boost is largely due to exercise's ability to improve circulation and blood flow to the brain. Elderly adults who engage in even low-intensity movements, such as cooking, cleaning, and gardening, have been shown to be better protected from memory and vocabulary losses than sedentary individuals of the same age.

The improvements in memory and concentration from exercise such as walking can be immediate. For instance, one University of Illinois Urbana-Champaign study showed that adults who performed cardiovascular exercise such as walking had an increased memory capacity and reaction time when completing a mental task 30 minutes later as opposed to nonexercisers and even those who only partook in strength-training exercises.

Sticking to your walking routine over a period of time has additional brain benefits as well. For instance, one study found that when sedentary individuals started an exercise routine for just 30 minutes three times per week, they were better able to perform mental tasks and had an increased memory after 12 weeks. One reason for this improvement is that long-term exercise is believed to boost *brain-derived neurotrophic factor,* or BDNF. This secreted protein is instrumental in the development of brain tissue and nerve connections in the areas of the brain that contribute to higher reasoning. Increasing this protein through exercise can then help to enhance this area of the brain, improving memory and concentration.

## How walking can ward off dementia

According to the Mayo Clinic, dementia is not a specific disease; rather, the term describes a group of symptoms that affect thinking and social abilities enough to interfere with daily functioning. Although many causes of dementia exist, Alzheimer's disease is the most common cause of progressive dementia. The World Health Organization (WHO) estimates 35.6 million individuals are affected by dementia worldwide. In addition, it's estimated that one in every eight older Americans suffers from Alzheimer's disease.

Risk factors for developing dementia are similar to those for heart disease and diabetes. Having an elevated blood pressure or high cholesterol levels can significantly increase your risk. Having a wide waistline or too much belly fat can up your odds as well. In fact, a study published in *Neurology* found that having a wide waistline tripled the risk for memory and thinking problems later in life for overweight individuals. And the same study found even individuals who were at a healthy body weight but carried too much visceral fat had double the risk for developing these problems as compared to individuals with less belly fat. Walking on a regular basis has been shown to lower body fat, shrink the waistline, and lower blood pressure and cholesterol levels — all factors that when reduced can also reduce the risk of dementia.

So how much walking is enough when it comes to the fight against dementia? One Italian study found that individuals ages 65 and older who burned 417 calories per week (which averages out to walking about 5 miles per week at a moderate pace) were 27 percent less likely to develop dementia compared to individuals of the same age who were sedentary. This averages out to walking just 1 mile five days per week! As you can see, with just a small amount of effort, you can fight numerous diseases as well as keep your brain sharp just by walking!

# Reaping the Physical Benefits of Walking

Do you wake up in the morning feeling stiff and sore? Does your back start to hurt throughout the day? Do you feel your flexibility and range of motion shortening as you age? If you answered "yes" to any of these questions, then walking can have a major impact on the way you feel and your physical appearance just as much as it can benefit your internal health.

If you want to keep your bones and joints healthy and young, you have to use them. And by using them, I mean you have to get them in motion with physical activity each day. The more often you move, the less stiff you feel. Moving your body through walking helps to move your muscles and joints through a complete range of motion, which improves your flexibility. In addition, the more you challenge your muscles, the stronger they'll become. Strong muscles can help to protect joints, which can help ward off joint disorders such as arthritis.

Walking also helps you to shed unwanted pounds and inches. As you get closer and closer to an ideal body weight, your joint health will improve. Even just a few extra pounds can increase the strain on your knees, hips, back, and feet. This extra pressure and strain increases the risk of cartilage breakdown, leading to pain and arthritic symptoms. And even just a few pounds makes a huge difference. For instance, for every pound of body weight you lose, you take about four pounds of pressure off your knees!

When it comes to exercise to improve your physical health, not all exercise is created equal. Sure, high-intensity exercises such as running may help torch calories, but they also place a great strain on joints and bones. This strain can result in injuries that bring on chronic pain. It can also lead to an accelerated breakdown of cartilage, which decreases the health of your joints. To protect your joints, low-impact exercise such as walking is your best bet. This type of exercise takes away the jarring and pounding caused by high-intensity exercises, allowing you to gain all the benefits of exercise without the downside of increased risk of injury or pain.

This section gives you the lowdown on how walking can increase your flexibility, improve your posture, and position you for better bone and joint health.

## How walking can increase flexibility

As you age, you lose range of motion and the flexibility of your joints. That is, of course, unless you work on keeping it. Regular stretching should be part of any exercise routine to increase flexibility and prevent injury (I show you the best stretches for your walking workout in Chapter 6). However, certain exercises, just by their nature, help to naturally increase flexibility. And walking is one such exercise.

Even without stretching before and after a walking workout (which is not recommended — a proper warm-up and cool-down are always your best options for a successful workout and injury prevention), the interaction of your legs, arms, core, and head while walking help to increase your flexibility. Taking long step helps to stretch your hip flexors. Walking uphill stretches your calf muscles. Swinging your arms while you walk helps to stretch your arms and shoulders.

The more often you walk, and the more you switch up your walking workout and walk in different areas (for example, walking uphill or hiking), the more you challenge your muscles and joints. Varying your walking workout also helps you take your joints through their full range of motion, increasing your overall flexibility.

## How walking can improve posture

Want to look younger than your biological age in a second? Stand up straight! Your posture, whether good or poor, can impact your appearance. Those who stand up tall and display good posture are most often seen as being younger and more vibrant. But posture does more than just impact your appearance. It can also have a significant impact on your overall health.

Poor posture, such as standing with a hunched back or rounded shoulders, can lead to breathing problems, joint pain, increased fall risk, and increased back pain. The more misaligned your posture is, the more misaligned your joints may become. And if your joints are misaligned, you're more likely to feel stiff and sore with every step you take. However, having proper posture keeps your whole body in alignment. From your neck all the way down to your knees and feet, your joints stay aligned and are therefore healthier overall.

Walking can help to improve posture, especially if you pay attention to it. As you increase the speed of your walk, your muscles have to work harder to keep you upright. These are the same muscles that you use to sit up tall and to carry yourself with good posture. Although walking by itself helps to strength these muscles, you also want to think about your posture as you walk. Avoid looking down at the ground or hunching over with your shoulders and back as you walk. Instead, keep your chin up and look in front of you instead of down. Keep your core tight and your shoulders down and back. This position helps to strength your muscles, allowing you to have good posture all day long.

In addition to monitoring your body positions, many helpful products are available on the market to help improve flexibility and posture, from resistance bands to fitness balls to back and posture braces. They're sold everywhere from big box retailers like Wayfair (who offers free shipping and free returns online) to specialty stores such as Sports Authority and www.gomoji.com. It's possible to improve posture and flexibility on your own; however, if you're struggling with these areas or want to make progress more quickly, using these types of products can help.

## How walking can improve bone and joint health

Bone and joint disease are quite prevalent in America. According to the CDC, one in five adults has been diagnosed with arthritis. In addition, 49.7 percent of adults age 65 years or older have arthritis. In fact, it's estimated that by 2030, 67 million Americans ages 18 years and older will be diagnosed with this condition. The National Osteoporosis Foundation estimates about 12 million people over the age of 50 have osteoporosis and another 40 million have low bone mass, putting them at risk for developing osteoporosis. By 2020, the prevalence of osteoporosis is expected to climb to 14 million cases along with 47 million cases of low bone mass. With this rise, it is estimated that about 40 percent of Caucasian women and 13 percent of Caucasian men over the age of 50 will experience at least one fracture due to low bone density in their lifetime, as those of Caucasian decent along with those of Asian decent are at a greater risk of osteoporosis.

When you look at these statistics, you see that a staggering number of people are impacted by bone and joint disease on a daily basis. These diseases can be crippling over time. However, by just increasing daily movement with walking, these diseases can be prevented, managed, or even reversed!

When it comes to bone health, it doesn't take much to decrease the risk of fractures. A Harvard Medical School study found that women who walked just four hours per week were as much as 41 percent less likely to suffer a hip fracture compared to those who walked only one hour per week. Walking is a weight-bearing exercise, which can help to strengthen and build bone. The more you walk, the stronger the bones in your hips and legs can become, helping to protect against fracture.

Joint pain can also be managed and decreased with regular walking. Partaking in low-impact exercise, such as walking, over a six-month period was found to decrease joint pain in arthritis sufferers by 25 percent and decrease stiffness by 16 percent. Why does walking help? When you exercise, you strengthen muscles. The stronger your muscles are around your joints, the less stress there is on your joints. For instance, research has shown that having weak muscles in the thigh can increase the risk of osteoarthritis in the knee. However, just small gains in strength in these muscles, which walking can help with, can significantly reduce the risk.

Back pain, which affects as many as seven out of ten Americans, can also be reduced with walking. A study published in *The Spine Journal* found that just one exercise session can reduce lower back pain by as much as 10 to 50 percent. Other research found that just a ten-minute walk on the treadmill was shown to lead to a significant reduction in back pain. So why does such a small amount of walking lead to such a big impact on back pain? There may be many reasons. Walking can help to strengthen back muscles, improve posture, and improve flexibility — all things that can lessen back pain. In addition, working large muscle groups, such as the muscles in the legs and core, helps to stimulate signals from large nerves to the brain. The signals from the larger nerves are thought to block pain signals coming from smaller nerves, so you literally feel less pain. In addition, the boost in "feel-good" brain chemicals, such as serotonin and endorphins, helps you to feel better and manage pain better.

# Walking at Any Age

One of the greatest benefits of walking is that it can be done by anyone, anywhere. From about the age of 1 on, you have learned how to walk. It's something you do every day. Because you're accustomed to walking, you don't need to learn any new skills or buy any fancy equipment. It's an activity you can already safely do. No matter how young or old you are, if you can walk, you can start to walk to shed pounds and gain health benefits.

Walking is superior to many other forms of exercise for a variety of reasons. For starters, it's a form of movement that comes naturally. It is cheap, effective, and can be done pretty much anywhere at anytime. But walking offers other benefits over other exercises as well. Because it's a low-impact form of exercise, it puts much less stress on your bones and joints. This stress reduction helps to cut down on the injury risk associated with exercise and allows you to partake in a form of exercise that is invigorating without being painful or taxing on your body.

When it comes to exercise in the fight against obesity as well as disease, the focus is shifting away from intensive, structured exercise and more toward being physically active every day. Walking fits perfectly into this mold. If you hate to go to the gym or have never exercised before, you can still increase the number of steps you take each day and boost your overall fitness and health. And when focusing on just increasing daily activity, you can see why walking can work at any age. Elderly people with limited mobility can still get up and walk around their home a few extra minutes per day. A child can walk with his parents around the neighborhood sightseeing while improving fitness. A busy mom can fit in a few ten-minute walks throughout the day. As you can see, walking can really work for almost anyone, at any age.

Keep in mind, rewarding yourself after a tough workout can also be a great way to stay motivated at any age. Think of various ways you can treat yourself for staying on track with your exercise goals. Maybe you want to reward yourself with a quiet night out away from the kids, or maybe you prefer a reward as simple as a hot bath. Even a nice massage, such as a foot massage after a walk, is a great way to reward yourself. There are many options ranging in price, from spas to at-home options. For instance, the Moji 360 Foot Massager from www.gomoji.com may be a great option to have at home for an invigorating foot massage whenever you need an instant, relaxing reward.

## *Adapting your walking routine over a lifetime*

Think about the ways you walk every day. Now think about the ways you walked as a child or as a young adult. Has the way in which you walk most days evolved as you've gotten older? No matter what your age, walking and being physically active daily provides your body with positive benefits. However, how you walk may transition over your lifetime.

As a child, you may have spent time walking with friends, walking while playing games, or even walking around your school building. As a young adult, you may have walked for fitness, gone for hikes, or walked around the mall while shopping. If you became a parent, you may have walked while chasing after your little ones or while performing household chores such as grocery shopping and cooking. Once retired, you may have started walking leisurely for fitness or to enjoy the day. Perhaps you walk while gardening or with a sport such as golf.

How you walk can vary from day to day depending on your schedule, preferences, and location. Your physical limitations and ability to walk may also impact how often you walk and the type of walking you do. For instance, someone suffering from arthritis of the knees isn't likely to power walk uphill; however, that same person can take a leisurely walk on a flat surface. Someone with chronic back pain may not be able to walk for more than a few minutes at a time. However, that person may be able to take brief walks multiple times per day to increase her activity level.

Your reasons for walking may also impact the type of walking you do. If you're focused on losing weight quickly, you may want to take longer, fast-paced walks. If you're walking to mostly reduce stress, you may find a stroll in the park is more your style. And even your style and duration of walking may vary from day to day based on your schedule and even your energy level.

Regardless of the type of walking you do, where you do it, or how intense you make it, the act of getting up and moving is all you need to gain the health and weight-loss benefits of walking. If your body limits you from taking long walks, a few brief walks can be just as beneficial. If you have joint pain, taking a long, slow walk can help you to shed pounds just as well as a fast-paced, short walk. All that matters is that you get up and get moving.

## Getting started at any age

Regardless of how old or young you are, the fact that you have picked up this book and started reading it shows that you are interested in starting a walking routine. As you think about how you can increase the amount of walking you do each day, ask yourself the following questions:

✔ What are my main goals for my walking routine?

✔ How am I already walking most days?

✔ How much time can I realistically devote to walking each day?

✔ How would I enjoy walking the most?

Using your answers to these questions, you can start to see what times of day may be best for you to walk, how much time you may be able to schedule each day for walking, and the type of walking that you would enjoy the most.

Remember, in order for you to be successful with an exercise routine such as walking, it needs to be enjoyable as well as practical.

Look at your current daily routine. Are there ways you can add in a few extra minutes of walking to increase your overall physical activity each day? For instance, perhaps you can park farther away at your office to increase the amount of steps it takes for you to go inside. At home, maybe you can carry the laundry in two trips instead of trying to juggle it all at once. As a family, perhaps you can take a walk after dinner and chat about your day instead of watching a television show. If you love TV, try getting up at the commercial breaks and walking instead of staying on the couch. Although these small amounts of movement don't seem like much, they can really add up. Just moving more throughout the day can increase the amount of calories you burn, boost your metabolism, and help you to shed pounds and inches.

# *Taking precautions later in life*

Later in life, it's more common to suffer from health conditions such as osteo-arthritis, osteoporosis, or even heart disease and diabetes. Every health condition presents your body with a unique set of challenges. These health conditions can also increase your risks as you look toward starting or chang-ing an exercise routine. For instance, with diabetes, foot care is essential, espe-cially when exercising, to prevent wounds that may not heal. Hypertension, or elevated blood pressure, must be monitored during exercise to prevent it from rising to a dangerous level. If you've been diagnosed with osteoporosis, you must take precautions against falls that could result in fractures.

When it comes to your health and your well-being, you can never be too cau-tious. Increasing your daily movement and steps generally does not require clearance by your physician. However, starting an exercise routine, such as walking for a set duration or at a higher intensity than you are accustomed to, may require a visit to your physician first. The American College of Sports Medicine (ACSM) recommends that you see your doctor before engaging in exercise if you have at least two of the following characteristics:

- You're a man older than 45 or a woman older than 55.
- You have a family history of heart disease before age 55 in men or age 65 in women.
- You're a smoker or quit smoking within the last six months.
- You haven't exercised for at least 30 minutes three days per week for three months or more.
- You are overweight or obese.
- You have high blood pressure or high cholesterol levels.
- You have diabetes or impaired glucose tolerance (sometimes referred to as prediabetes).

Although not mentioned on the ACSM precaution list, those with arthritis or osteoporosis should also see their physician before starting a walking routine to discuss the best walking techniques for protecting your joint and bone health. Seeing your physician before starting your walking rou-tine ensures that you can get started safely with a routine that will improve your health without the risk of injury or worsening any current health conditions.

It's very important to incorporate braces, wraps, ointments, and other products into your routine if you've been injured or to prevent injury if you are at a high risk of injury. For instance, those with preexisting injuries or diseases such as arthritis may benefit from using these products. You should consult your doctor for specific recommendations. Most drug stores sell basic products, and there are some very good specialty stores whose product lines are more tailored to each unique injury and body type. I list and describe some unique products that you may find helpful on my website as well.

## Maximizing your walking workout at any age

Although the intensity and type of walking you may participate in will most likely change and evolve throughout your lifespan, you can maximize your walking workout to increase your calorie burn, boost metabolism, and shed pounds at any age. Although I address these techniques in greater depth in Chapter 11, I outline them for you here so you can begin to think about how you may be able to incorporate them into your daily routine.

- **Keep good posture.** Making sure to keep your head up, your shoulders pulled back and down, and your core tight during exercise not only improves your form, but also activates more muscles during your walk. The harder your muscles work, the more calories they burn.

- **Increase daily activity as well as scheduled exercise.** Adding a structured walk, such as a 30-minute walk daily, is a great way to lose weight and get in shape. However, some research has found that individuals who perform a structured workout, such as an hour at the gym, but have a mostly sedentary day otherwise, burn less calories than people who are generally up on their feet most of the day. So do both! Schedule that walk, but make sure you aren't sitting the rest of the day. If you have a desk job, get up and stretch or walk around every hour or so.

- **Add interval training.** Adding intervals to your walking routine can torch calories as well as boost fitness more rapidly than working out at a consistent intensity level for the duration of the workout. How do intervals work? Take a 20-minute walk, for instance: You walk at a moderate 3-miles-per-hour (mph) pace for five minutes, then for one minute you bump up the pace to walk as quickly as you can (for instance, 4 mph), then you bring your speed back down again for five minutes, and repeat over and over again for the duration of the workout. This type of technique helps to elevate your heart rate and keep it elevated for most of your workout, burning more calories.

- **Power up your walk.** Power walking can have many different meanings, but essentially it just means walking at a brisk pace. If you typically walk at a pace where you can comfortably carry on a conversation, this is more of a leisurely walk. By pushing yourself to pump up the pace to where you can still speak but not carry on a full conversation, you are elevating your heart rate and therefore your calorie expenditure.

✔ **Don't be scared of an incline.** Walking at an incline, such as walking uphill, can help you to challenge your muscles and boost your calorie burn. If you tend to walk on a flat surface, choosing a different terrain can help turn up your workout and speed up your results.

✔ **Adding weights.** Adding weights such as hand weights to your walking workout can increase the amount of calories you burn per minute. According to the American Council on Exercise, people who wear light weights during exercise burn approximately 5 to 15 percent more calories on average than people who do not. The same can be said for adding resistance to your walking workout, such as pushing a stroller. This tactic increases the challenge to your muscles and therefore boosts your calorie burn and your results. If you have any pre-existing medical conditions, joint issues, prior injuries, or have been diagnosed with osteopenia or osteoporosis, make sure to ask your physician before adding weights if this form of exercise is appropriate for you and any precautions you must take.

# Combining Daily Activity with Workout Walking

When it comes to walking, there are plenty of ways to work it into your day. Walking doesn't just have to be something that you schedule a time to do, such as taking a 30-minute walk at lunchtime. In fact, it may be more beneficial to your health and waistline to think about incorporating movement and walking into all of your daily activities, rather than just scheduling it in for a certain amount of time. Not only does it make walking less of a chore and something that's more a part of your daily life, but it may actually help you reach your weight-loss goals faster.

Many research studies suggest that daily active living, such as taking the stairs over the elevator or standing while talking on the phone versus sitting, can be even healthier than hitting the gym. Many times, going to the gym for an hour may leave you feeling tired and sore. This outcome may result in you being less active the rest of the day, cancelling out the calorie benefit you burned off at the gym. In fact, people who are generally active during the day have been found to burn more calories overall than those who go to the gym but are mostly sedentary the remainder of the day.

When you think of walking, there are essentially two ways to incorporate it into your day:

- ✔ **Walking for exercise:** You schedule a time of day and walk within a certain time frame or for a certain duration continuously.

- ✔ **Walking for daily activity:** You increase your overall daily movement per day by parking farther away, taking the stairs more often, or standing versus sitting.

Both forms of walking are great for health, but to achieve your weight-loss and health goals in the quickest way possible, a combination of the two is your best bet. Scheduling in a walk during the day helps to boost metabolism and strengthen muscles, whereas increasing your overall movement helps to maximize your calorie burn throughout the day.

## Managing your weight

When it comes to losing weight and keeping it off, it's all about taking in fewer calories than you burn. However, diet alone doesn't always lead to successful weight loss. Regular exercise helps you burn more calories throughout the day as well as boost metabolism. This means that your body is burning more calories overall, allowing you to take in more calories without a change in weight.

If you have a slow metabolism, you can only cut back on calories so much before you're feeling hungry much of the day. In addition, reducing your calorie intake too far can actually further slow metabolism. In order to make weight loss easier, burning more calories through exercise is essential.

Take a look at this example. It takes approximately 3,500 calories to burn off one pound of fat. Sally is a woman in her 60s who has a short stature. Her sex, age, and height all lead to her having a slower metabolism. Sally, on average, burns about 1,300 calories per day at rest. Eating less than 1,200 calories per day can slow her metabolism, which Sally doesn't want to happen. So, if Sally eats exactly 1,200 calories per day, without any exercise, she has a deficit of 100 calories per day. This means it will take her 35 days to lose just 1 pound. This is doable, but of course, Sally, just like you, wants to see results faster than that.

The benefits of exercise and daily activity can have a big impact on Sally and her weight-loss efforts. If Sally starts to track her daily steps and increases them from walking 4,000 steps per day to 10,000 steps per day, she will be walking an extra 3 miles per day (every 2,000 steps equals just about one mile of walking). Because walking a mile burns about 100 calories, that boosts

Sally's overall calorie expenditure from only 1,300 calories per day to 1,600. Just with this little change she will lose closer to 1/2 to 1 pound per week instead of just 1 pound per month.

Now if, on top of this daily increase in steps, Sally decides to schedule a three-mile walk three days per week, she'll burn an additional 900 calories per week, or an extra pound per month. Using this example, you can see how quickly those extra steps and walks add up when it comes to shedding pounds and inches!

# Preventing and managing disease

Just like in the preceding example of Sally, the more you move, the more it benefits your body. Increased walking helps you to achieve a healthier body weight, which alone decreases disease risk. But just moving more can also help to lower blood pressure, blood sugar, and cholesterol levels. In addition, added physical activity can help to decrease joint pain and build bone mass. But in order to gain these benefits, you don't have to devote a set amount of time to walking.

Cumulative exercise and movement is just as effective for weight management and health as large chunks of exercise. If you were to walk for ten minutes three times per day, that would be just as beneficial to your overall health as walking for 30 minutes at once. Sometimes breaking up exercise into these intervals can be even more beneficial. For instance, say you take a 10-minute walk at breakfast, lunch, and dinner. Well, if one day your schedule gets too busy in the evening and you can't fit in your usual walk, you'll still have walked 20 minutes that day. Now, if you usually walk 30 minutes at once after dinner, skipping this walk would mean not walking at all.

# Tracking and increasing your daily movement

When it comes to increasing your movement per day, tracking steps is the easiest way to go about determining your level of activity. There are many wonderful new products and technologies that help you easily track your fitness and diet progress.

### Choosing a tool for your needs and budget

Before you take the plunge and make a significant investment in some of the higher-end fitness technologies, you can start out with a simple pedometer, which is a tool that tracks the number of steps a person takes while walking. It's generally worn on the waist belt of your pants to give you the most accurate measurement. When tracking steps, it's helpful to know that 2,000 steps per day is equal to just about a mile of walking. One of my favorite pedometers is Accusplit (www.accusplit.com), but there are many options that offer a variety of features. You can see a full list and review the various features of each on my website.

If you really want to go high-tech with your fitness tracking, wearable technology is the hottest trend, and it makes your tracking effortless. You can find stylish pedometers and heart rate monitors. I highly recommend the investment, which can range from as little as $10 up to $300–400. On the high end, a must-have is an activity tracker wristband sold by Fitbit. Many other wristband trackers, which can track daily steps and overall physical activity, are available as well; all are very fashionable, and all offer similar benefits, including tracking calories burned, steps taken, time walked, miles walked, and even your sleep patterns. You can wear them 24/7 to get a really accurate readout of your calorie burn to fitness ratio to help maximize your weight-loss progress.

Some of these activity trackers automatically sync wirelessly over Bluetooth and are also integrated with a digital scale and/or an app showing your walk on a map that you can post to Facebook. They typically offer a website where you can access and view your progress anytime, anywhere. I talk about these products, which trackers work with what, and more on my website. You can find them at big box retailers or specialty stores that have a wider array of selections, such as www.heartratemonitors.com.

### Getting your steps in every day

The ACSM recommends that everyone aim to walk at least 10,000 steps per day for general health. This is the number of steps research has found you need to burn enough calories to reduce the risk of obesity and chronic disease. However, just increasing the number of steps you take per day will make a difference in your health and your weight, even if you can't yet reach this goal. To increase your steps, use the following guidelines to get started:

- ✔ Wear your pedometer from the time you get up in the morning until the time you go to bed for at least three days to get a baseline of the average number of steps you usually take.

- ✔ After you know your baseline number of steps (for example 4,000 steps per day), increase the amount of steps you take daily by 10 to 20 percent per week. (Based on the example of 4,000 steps per day, you could try to increase your daily steps by 400 to 800 steps. After doing this for one week, aim to add another 400 to 800 steps each day.)

- ✔ Continue to increase your steps each week until you reach at least 10,000 steps per day.

# Chapter 3

# How Walking Sheds Pounds

**C**onsider this: Just walking a little more each day will lead to pounds and inches falling off. Does it sound too simple? It may seem that way, but it's really true. By increasing the amount of walking you do each and every day, you can start to reach your long-term weight-loss goals, flatten your stomach, and tone and tighten all the muscles in your body. And it truly is as simple as placing one foot in front of the other.

If you've tried over and over again to lose weight and it just hasn't worked, you may need to reevaluate what you've been doing.

If you've tried to watch what you eat but haven't given any thought to increasing your activity, that may be part of the problem. In order to lose weight and keep it off, you must, of course, eat a healthy diet rich in whole foods (I show you just how to fuel your walking workout and torch additional pounds and inches through diet in Chapters 7 and 8). But if you only watch your diet and do nothing else, weight loss may plateau or not happen at all. On the flip side, if you increase your activity level, but also eat more, you won't lose weight either. The real solution is to eat healthfully and move more to lose weight and keep it off for good. Adjusting one without the other rarely results in successful weight loss.

# Walking: The Cheap and Easy Way to Lose Weight

Walking is the number one form of exercise for good reason. Over 100 million Americans walk each and every day to boost health and lose weight. These people start walking and continue to do it for one reason: It works!

Walking really does help you shed pounds and keep them off. Just look at the statistics from the National Weight Control Registry, which is one of the largest weight-loss studies ever conducted. This registry, which has over 10,000 members enrolled, studies the behaviors of individuals who have lost at least 30 pounds and have kept the weight off for at least one year. On average, the members of this registry have lost 66 pounds and have maintained that loss for 5.5 years. So how have they been so successful at not just losing weight, but actually keeping it off? The overwhelming majority walk! Ninety-four percent have increased their overall physical activity, with the most frequently reported form of activity being walking. In fact, 54 percent of the women in the registry report walking a mile or more per day. So, as you can see, walking certainly seems to be working for them, and it can work for you too!

So why does walking work so well for so many people? For starters, it's cheap, it's easy, you don't have to learn any skills to do it, and you can really do it anywhere. The easier something is to do, the more likely you are to do it. And that's really the secret to walking for weight loss — it's too simple not to do!

## The impact walking has on weight loss

As I mention in Chapter 2, you have to burn approximately 3,500 calories to lose one pound of body weight. That sounds like a lot, especially when you consider how quickly calories can add up, especially if you aren't eating the right types of foods. If you're thinking that it would also take a lot of movement to burn that amount of calories, you're right. In order to burn 3,500 calories, you'd need to walk about 35 miles at a moderate pace. That's quite a distance! In fact, that would be like walking a full marathon and then walking nine more miles for fun after you finish. When you look at it that way, it can seem almost impossible (not to mention exhausting!) to burn off a pound just by walking.

The good news is that you don't have to strap on a pair of sneakers and hit the road for 35 miles to start shedding pounds. You don't even have to walk ten or even five miles at a time. All you have to do is start moving a bit more throughout the day. Think about exercise in the same way you think about eating for weight loss. Yes, we all know that consuming an entire pizza in one sitting will most likely send the scale in the wrong direction. But what if you just pick on little bites of cookie throughout the day? It seems harmless, right? And you barely even notice you're doing it. But after a week of picking here and there, you may see that you've gained a few ounces or even a pound or two and wonder what happened. You probably don't feel like you over-ate at all. You may have even thought you were losing weight. But those tiny little bites here and there really add up over the course of a full day.

Just like eating tiny bites of food over and over again all day long can result in taking in way more calories than you realize, taking tiny steps here and there throughout the day can help you to burn a lot more calories than you may think possible. Begin to wear a pedometer to track and count your steps. On average, 2,000 steps of walking equals about one mile. One mile of walking at a moderate pace burns about 100 calories.

Consider a typical day for Peter, who has a desk job. Peter wakes up in the morning, takes a shower, eats a quick breakfast, and then sits in the car for an hour driving to work. He gets to work a little late, so he parks as close to the entry door as possible. He rushes to his desk where he sits for the next eight hours working on his computer and taking phone calls. He then sits in the car on the way home, has dinner, watches TV, and goes to bed.

On a typical day, Peter walks about 2,500 steps. Now, look at just how much adding a few steps here and there can increase the amount of calories Peter burns each day:

- When Peter gets to work, he finds the farthest parking spot, so he has to walk farther to get into his building (500 steps).

- At work, every time Peter takes a phone call, he stands up and paces versus sitting in his chair (3,000 steps).

- On his lunch break, Peter takes a brisk, 10-minute stroll around his office building (1,000 steps).

- At the end of the workday, Peter walks back to his car, which he parked farther away when he arrived (500 steps).

- At home while watching TV, Peter gets up during the commercial breaks and walks versus sitting on the couch (1,500 steps).

Just by making these small changes, and without having to schedule additional time into his day, Peter has added an extra 6,500 steps or an extra 3.25 miles of walking! As a result, he burns an additional 325 calories per day. If he makes no other changes to his diet or his exercise level, just by adding these steps he will start to lose almost three pounds per month, or 34 pounds in a year! So you can see just how much these small steps really add up!

# Why walking may be the best exercise for weight management

As noted earlier in this chapter, walking is by far the most commonly used exercise of people who are successful at losing weight and keeping it off. But why is walking the best exercise for weight loss? Compare it to some other forms of exercise to see:

- ✔ **Walking versus running:** Although running may burn more calories per minute, it also results in increased wear and tear on your bones and joints. For individuals with joint pain or arthritis, running for more than a minute or two at a time may be impossible due to pain. In addition, injury risk is higher with running as compared to walking. If you experience joint pain or suffer an injury, you're unlikely to be able to keep up with your running routine. With walking, joint pain is limited thanks to walking's low-impact nature, which means you can walk more often and for longer distances with less impact on your body.

- ✔ **Walking versus bike riding:** Riding a bike can take some of the pressure off your joints; however, in order to ride a bike, you need a bike — either a regular bike or a stationary bike. You also need access to a safe road to bike on or to a space in your home or at a gym to ride a stationary bike. Because biking requires more equipment and can't be done anywhere at any time like walking, it's less convenient. When it comes to starting an exercise routine, you want it to be as easy as possible for you to stick with. Biking opens the door for excuses, such as the weather isn't nice, the road is too busy, you don't feel like driving to the gym, and so on. With walking, whether you're home, at work, or out with friends, there's always an opportunity to get in a few extra steps.

- ✔ **Walking versus swimming:** Swimming is a great low-impact exercise, especially for those with joint pain and arthritis. The downside of swimming is that it requires access to a pool, lake, or ocean. In addition, with swimming, you need time to put on a bathing suit as well as dry off afterward. If you're looking to squeeze in a quick workout on your lunch break, jumping in the pool may not be realistic based on the extra time needed to change and dry off.

- ✔ **Walking versus group exercises:** Depending on the form of group exercise or classes you choose, it may be low- or high-impact. Higher-impact fitness classes may torch more calories, but as with running, they carry a higher risk of injury and joint pain. Fitness classes also require a space to perform them, whether you have a room in your home or you travel to a gym. They also entail following a DVD or taking a class, which involves a cost. Group exercise also can't be done anywhere as easily as walking can.

You may feel embarrassed performing dance moves for ten minutes on your lunch break at work or on the sidelines of your child's soccer game, whereas no one would think you looked out of place walking around your office or the soccer field.

As you can see, when compared to almost any other exercise, there's no getting around the convenience and accessibility of walking. The easier you make it to fit exercise into your day, the easier it will be to stick with your exercise routine. That's why walking works so well: It's simple, it's inexpensive, and it can be done anywhere!

# Walking Your Way to Results

When it comes to the battle of the bulge, one of the main benefits walking has over other forms of exercise is its ability to be done often. Some exercise forms, such as running, take a large toll on your body. If you were to go for multiple runs over the course of a day, you'd no doubt feel it in your knees and back the following day. If you woke up too sore, you'd most likely be unable to exercise the next day, which would then lessen the amount of calories you could burn throughout the week. However, because walking can be done leisurely or briskly with a limited impact on your body, you can take two 30-minute walks one day and wake up feeling rejuvenated and energized the next day, allowing you to continue to be active day after day. Because walking allows you to do it easily and more often, it can be more effective at helping you shed pounds and inches as well as keep them off.

The consistency that walking allows is what makes it such a powerful weight-loss tool. In order to lose weight and keep it off, you must have a calorie deficit every day. If you've started an exercise routine in the past, I'm sure you are no stranger to having some days where you just don't feel like exercising or your joints and muscles need a day to rest. With walking, even if you have a day where you can't seem to talk yourself into taking a brisk power walk, you can still increase your daily steps without putting too much effort into it. By increasing your steps, even on your days off from structured exercise, you are still burning more calories and challenging your muscles. All of this results in an elevated metabolism and an increase in total calorie expenditure throughout the day, promoting weight loss. If in the past you were unsuccessful at losing pounds and inches with exercise, ask yourself if you were consistent with your exercise routine. If you had not been, that was most likely the reason for the lack of progress. However, following any of the walking routines in this book will allow you to become consistent with exercise day after day, providing you with fast and effective results that will last. In the following section, I outline for you the impact walking can have on your overall body composition and just how it helps you to shed body fat.

## *The impact of walking on body composition*

Not only can walking help you to shed pounds, but it can also make sure you lose the right type of weight. Changing your diet to lose weight without adding any exercise can result in losing muscle mass as well as fat. Muscle is what makes up the majority of your metabolism. So if you lose muscle, you burn fewer calories throughout the day. You may reach your goal weight but actually burn less calories than you did before you started losing weight.

To see what this could mean for you, take a look at research conducted on seniors following a weight-loss program. One group of seniors exercised while dieting, and another group followed only a diet program. Although both groups lost similar amounts of weight, the group that did not exercise lost three times more muscle mass. In addition, the exercising group was found to increase their fat-burning ability by twice as much as the non-exercisers. A loss in muscle like the one found in this study can make keeping weight off very difficult. This is one of the main reasons why adding exercise, such as walking, is so critical not just to losing weight, but also to maintaining that weight loss.

One of the most dangerous types of fat in your body is visceral fat, otherwise known as belly fat. As I mention in Chapter 1, having a wide waistline is the main criteria used to determine whether you have too much of this deadly fat. Having excess belly fat is not just damaging to your silhouette in clothing, but it can also increase your risk for a number of diseases. For instance, having excess belly fat has been associated with an increased risk for heart disease, diabetes, dementia, and even certain cancers! Diet can certainly help you to shed this unwanted fat, but exercise, such as walking, helps you to lose this weight more quickly and keep it off.

To see the dramatic impact walking can have on belly fat, take a look at one study conducted at Wake Forest University Baptist Medical Center. This study looked at two groups of women: one group who dieted for weight loss without walking and one group that walked one to two miles just three times per week. Even though both groups were able to lose weight, the group that walked a few times per week shrank their belly fat cells by 18 percent over a four-month period. And what happened to the nonwalking group? Their belly fat cells remained unchanged! So even though weight came off, the most dangerous source of body fat remained unchanged without walking.

Even if you make no change to your diet at all, walking can help improve your body composition for the better. By walking briskly for one hour per day without changing eating habits, research found a 20 percent reduction in belly fat over a three-month period. So regardless of whether or not you're changing your diet to lose weight, adding walking to your regular routine helps you to gain muscle, shed belly fat, and lose those stubborn inches and pounds for good.

# *Walking to speed results*

Walking by itself, no matter how you choose to do it, can help you to burn more calories and shed body fat. However, there are certain ways you can walk that will help you to increase the amount of calories you burn per minute, increase muscles mass, boost metabolism, and see results faster. I outline these techniques in more detail in Chapter 11; however, you may want to give some thought to which of these techniques, if any, will work best for you:

- ✔ **Tracking steps in addition to taking structured walks:** Using a pedometer to track and increase your steps each day can be a great way to help you boost your overall calorie expenditure. The same can be said of taking a structured walk daily. However, if you walk for an hour on your lunch break but then are sedentary the rest of the day, you may not burn as many calories as you think. If you track and increase your steps each day, you may boost your calorie burn, but you may not gain the health and metabolism benefits of structured exercise. The solution is to utilize both techniques by wearing a pedometer every day and planning to go for a walk of at least 30 minutes in duration a few times per week.

- ✔ **Weighing yourself down:** Adding any form of resistance to your walking workout challenges your muscles. When you challenge your muscles, you gain an increase in muscle mass, which also helps to boost metabolism. The more muscle you have, the more calories you burn each and every day, even when at rest. In addition, a more muscular frame makes weight maintenance easier as well. Using resistance bands, dumbbells, or even the resistance from pushing a stroller are all ways to boost muscle mass and metabolism.

- ✔ **Changing up your terrain:** Your body is an amazing machine and it quickly adapts to challenges. As great as this is, if you perform the same workout day in and day out, your body will become accustomed to it. When your body is used to an exercise, it becomes easier for you, which means it no longer challenges your muscles or cardiovascular system as much as it once did. This results in fewer calories being burned during the workout as well as fewer gains in muscle strength and size. To prevent this, change up your walking terrain every few weeks. If you walk on a flat surface, switch to an incline such as walking uphill. If you walk on a treadmill, switch up your workout by taking it outside. The more you vary your workout, the more it will continue to challenge your body and speed your results.

- ✔ **Varying your speed:** Just as your body can become accustomed to your workout terrain, it can become accustomed to the speed at which you walk. Walking at the same speed day after day fails to provide much of a challenge to your body, and you burn fewer calories and shed less fat. To prevent this, work on mixing up your speed. If you usually walk at a leisurely pace where you can carry on a conversation easily, pick up your speed to power walk and walk as briskly as you can. You can also incorporate interval training, where you walk at a slower speed for a few minutes and then walk as quickly as you can for a set period of time, repeating this pattern throughout your workout. Little changes like this can bring you big results in a short period of time!

# Reducing Your Appetite with Exercise

In addition to the metabolism-boosting benefits of walking and the increased calorie expenditure walking offers, walking may help you to shed pounds in other ways. One way is by impacting your appetite.

Vigorous exercise, such as running, may suppress appetite for about an hour after completion. However, this benefit is short-lived, as appetite may then increase after this period of time. If you work hard to burn a large amount of calories during exercise only to feel ravenous and eat them all back — plus more — later on, you may feel like you're spinning your wheels when it comes to weight loss. That's where walking can help.

A study out of Brigham Young University found that exercise, specifically walking, may have an appetite-reducing effect on the body. These researchers found that subjects produced a lower brain response to food images on days when they performed a 45-minute, brisk walk in the morning as opposed to days when they didn't walk. Other research has shown that aerobic exercise, such as walking, may impact the release of ghrelin and peptide YY, two hormones that are key to your body's appetite regulation. It appears that aerobic exercise, such as walking, has a larger impact on suppressing appetite than nonaerobic exercise, such as weight lifting.

What does this research mean for you? Taking brisk walks throughout the day may help to take your mind off of food. In addition, walking may help your body to better process appetite hormones, allowing you to feel less hungry throughout the day and to feel fuller sooner when eating. All of these benefits can result in consuming fewer calories, which can help to speed weight-loss results.

## Walking away the cravings

Walking can impact more than just your appetite. Food cravings, such as that late-night ice cream craving or that midday desire for a salty snack, can be weight-loss sabotages. If you often experience food cravings, you know just how difficult they can be to overcome, especially if you are tired or stressed. If you've tried everything to overcome food cravings and haven't been successful, you may want to give walking a try!

A new study published in *Appetite* found that just a short bout of walking (only 15 minutes) was found to significantly reduce cravings for chocolate. Previous studies also found that moderate walking on a treadmill, at a pace considered brisk but not tiring, also helped individuals to overcome cravings for chocolate and pass by the stuff when tempted. One of the reasons walking may help to curb these cravings is its ability to increase dopamine in the body. This hormone provides you with an increased sense of pleasure and satisfaction (the same way you may feel after indulging in a chocolate bar). Because walking alone helps to improve your pleasure signals, you may not feel the desire to use food to boost this hormone as well.

It may not be all about hormone production when it comes to fighting cravings either. If you don't get enough sleep and walk around chronically tired, you have a higher likelihood of experiencing food cravings throughout the day. Studies have shown that individuals who get poor sleep tend to consume more calories and often crave higher-calorie, lower nutrient-dense food such as candy and sweets. Because walking has been shown to improve both quality and quantity of sleep, a more-rested you may have fewer food cravings to battle.

## *Managing post-workout hunger*

Many times, especially if you are new to exercise, you may experience an increase in appetite. If you aren't careful, this effect can sabotage your weight-loss efforts. As research has shown, walking may have less of an impact on post-workout-induced hunger than other forms of exercise, but it can still happen. How much your appetite increases after exercise can be based on many factors, including the following:

- ✔ The timing and balance of your meals and snacks
- ✔ Your hydration levels
- ✔ The intensity of your workout
- ✔ The duration of your workout

Typically, a workout that is higher in intensity and duration results in a larger boost in appetite after completion.

If you find that your appetite is constantly higher after walking, you can try a few strategies to improve your situation:

- ✔ Slightly decrease the intensity of your walk by walking a bit slower or at less of an incline. You can increase the length of the walk at a lower intensity, which may help to better control appetite.

- ✔ Make sure you stay well hydrated. You should drink an extra 8 to 10 ounces of water for every 30 minutes of walking.

- ✔ Space out your workout during the day. For instance, instead of walking for one hour, walk for 20 minutes three times during the day.

- ✔ Plan to have a snack or meal within 30 minutes of completing your workout. Flip to Chapter 7 for more details on the best nutrients before and after your workout to regulate appetite and burn fat.

# The Movement and Mood Connection

The more you move, the better you feel. When you feel better, you want to keep moving. The more you keep moving, the easier it is to lose weight and keep it off. See how that works? But the reverse is true too. If you feel down or tired, talking yourself into moving can be hard. And the less you move, the more fatigued you become. The more fatigued you are, the harder it is to get motivated to eat well, cook, fight food cravings, and so on. As you can see, exercise isn't just about the calorie boost when it comes to losing weight and keeping it off. It provides much, much more!

One of the biggest benefits walking offers when it comes to weight management is its ability to lift mood. If you're someone who eats to reward yourself or are a stress eater, you can see just why this is so important. If you tend to turn to food when you're emotional, you are eating for reasons other than hunger. Regardless of whether you're hungry or full at the time, you're eating with your mind rather than your stomach. If you are able to gain a better hold of your emotions, lift your spirits, and manage stress, you'll be better able to control your food intake and therefore your weight.

## Improving your mood with exercise

Moving your body helps to boost circulation. This increased circulation then brings blood and oxygen to all the cells of your body, helping you to feel rejuvenated and energized. In addition, exercise can help to release endorphins, those feel-good chemicals in the brain. These chemicals signal a sense of calmness to your body and decrease stress levels. The boost in energy as well as the lifted mood exercise promotes can have a large impact on the food choices you make.

Although all exercise may help to boost mood and energy, some exercises have a greater impact than others.

Walking has been found to be an exercise associated with the greatest impact on mood and energy. In fact, walking, as opposed to an exercise such as running, has been found to make exercisers feel better not only after they complete their walk, but also while they are walking as well. And if you feel great while walking, don't you think you'll want to do it more often? One of the greatest benefits of walking is that it feels good to do it. If you feel great after a run, but it's hard to talk yourself into doing it because your joints ache while you run, you're not likely to stick with that exercise program. However, an exercise that makes you feel good while doing it as well as afterward is one you'll stick with for life. And that's walking!

Even small amounts of walking can really add up. Physical activity, even in small increments, has been shown to increase production of those feel-good neurotransmitters in the brain. Walking, when preformed on a regular basis, has also been shown to increase self-confidence and even lower the symptoms associated with anxiety and mild depression. If you don't have time to fit in a long walk, take a few minutes to go for a short, brisk walk. You can even break from your day for just a few minutes to stretch and fit in a few steps — it all adds up!

## How mood impacts weight

Think about the last time you woke up feeling well rested and like you had all the energy in the world. What did you do that day? Did you spring out of bed and have the ambition to accomplish a large number of tasks that day? Did you find yourself moving on your feet more because you were being so productive? Were you more inclined to exercise because you had so much energy? Did you eat healthier foods because you craved them over junk food? Did you have the energy you needed to shop for food and cook rather than call for takeout? Chances are at least a few of these things happened for you on such an energetic day. And when you are able to be more active, eat healthier, and feel better about yourself, you're more apt to continue to make healthy behavior choices.

As you can see, how you feel can have just as much impact on your body weight as what you eat. When you feel good, you want to continue to feel that way, so you tend to repeat behaviors that make you feel good. If walking boosts your energy and your mood, you tend to keep walking. This boost in mood helps you to have more energy to prepare healthy foods. These foods then also make you feel even better, so you're more inclined to continue to eat them, and the list goes on and on.

# Stress and Walking

Stress affects everyone in different ways. When you are under stress, your mind, body, and behavior are all impacted. A small amount of stress can actually be beneficial. Stress can make you more alert, make you more productive, and even boost your energy level — but only in small amounts.

At a certain point, stress stops becoming helpful and starts to become harmful. In fact, stress can creep up on you over time until it can start to feel almost normal; however, it can still be damaging to your health. You may not notice how much it's affecting you until it starts to take a toll on your health.

Everyone is different in terms of the amount of stress they can handle. One person may find a certain situation very stressful whereas another person may thrive in the same environment. What's important is that you recognize the signs and symptoms of stress overload in your own self, so you can identify when you are under too much stress and when it's time to take control of it. When you are under too much stress, you may start to notice changes in your mood, behavior, and even your health. For instance, you may find yourself

- ✔ Eating more or less than normal
- ✔ Feeling anxious or irritable
- ✔ Sleeping too much or too little
- ✔ Feeling overwhelmed
- ✔ Displaying physical symptoms like gastrointestinal upset or muscle aches

The body doesn't distinguish between physical and psychological threats. So when you are under emotional stress, such as meeting a work deadline, your body responds in the same way it would to a physical stress, such as running away from a predator. When your body faces a stressful situation, it releases stress hormones such as cortisol and adrenaline. If you find yourself under chronic stress day after day, long-term exposure to these stress hormones being elevated in the body can lead to serious health problems such as elevated blood pressure, increased belly fat, and even heart disease and diabetes.

You may feel like the stress in your life is beyond your control, but you can always control the way you respond to it. By implementing stress-busting behaviors into your daily routine, you can take control of your stress levels before they take control of you.

## *Walking to reduce stress levels*

Exercise is one of the best physical stress-reduction techniques. In almost no time at all, regular exercise can help to reduce stress hormones, lower heart rate, and have you feeling relaxed and energized.

Walking is one of the best exercises for stress reduction because it can be done at any intensity level and, being low impact, provides little physical stress to the body. By walking you can

- ✔ Improve blood flow to your brain, bringing additional sugars and oxygen that may be needed when you are concentrating intensely.

- ✔ Reduce mental stress brought on by intense concentration. During periods of high-intensity focus, the neurons of your brain function more intensely and build up toxic waste products that can cause a sense of "foggy thinking." By walking, you can speed the flow of blood through your brain, moving these waste products faster and allowing you to clear your mind.

- ✔ Release endorphins into your bloodstream, giving you a feeling of happiness and positively affecting your overall sense of well-being.

The benefits of walking are long-lived as well. Research has found that walking can reduce anxiety for a full day thanks to the boost of serotonin and dopamine it provides. Walking has also been shown to ease muscle tension and provide a break from mental stressors, allowing it to have a relaxing effect on both your mind and your body.

## *Reducing stress to improve body weight and composition*

If you've been under a large amount of stress for a period of time, you may have noticed that your body weight has stayed about the same while your waistline has increased. Why has this happened?

Emotional and physical stressors on your body can lead to the release of stress hormones, including cortisol and adrenaline. These stress hormones then mobilize fatty acid stores from all areas of your body such as your thighs and arms. If these fatty acids are not used by your body (and when you are under emotional stress, your energy needs do not increase, leaving the majority unused) they get redeposited. And where do the majority of these fat stores go? They go right to your midsection! This widens your waistline while increasing dangerous belly fat and increasing your risk of disease.

As you can see, high stress levels can start to impact body composition and increase the amount of belly fat you carry. In addition, stress can often impact eating habits, resulting in further weight gain as well.

High stress levels may increase food cravings for sweets or salty foods. Sometimes stress can increase the desire to eat for reasons other than hunger, such as grabbing a bag of chips to unwind after a long day or sitting down with ice cream to boost your mood after a fight with a friend. When you eat for reasons other than hunger, you typically consume too much of the wrong types of foods. This increase in calories then leads to an increase in body weight. However, incorporating behaviors into your day that can help to decrease stress, such as walking, can fight against stress-related weight gain.

## *Other techniques to reduce stress*

Although walking itself helps to lower stress levels, certain techniques can help to maximize the stress-reduction efforts of your workout. As I mention in Chapter 6 and describe in more detail in Chapter 7, stretching during your warm-up and cool-down for your walking routine is vital in helping to protect you against injury. However, in addition, stretching offers other benefits as well.

One of the benefits of stretching is its ability to help reduce stress levels. Stretching exercises help to relieve stress as they get the blood flowing throughout your body. By improving circulation and increasing flexibility, stretching helps to cut down on stress by bringing vital oxygen and nutrients to cells and relieving muscle tension. Stretching also helps to stimulate receptors in the nervous system that decrease the production of stress hormones, further adding to its stress-lowering abilities.

The way in which you walk may also help to reduce stress. A study conducted by the University of Missouri-Columbia found higher intensity exercise helped to lower stress and anxiety levels more than less intensive exercise. Walking allows you to make your workout as intense or as easy as you like. When managing stress, try incorporating high-intensity interval training into your walking routine to cut stress levels the most. To do this, walk at your normal pace for five minutes. Then, walk as quickly as you can (or walk up as high an incline as you can) for one minute and then return to your original speed. Repeat these interval changes in speed or incline throughout the duration of your workout for the most effective stress reduction.

# Part II
# Preparing and Fueling Your Body

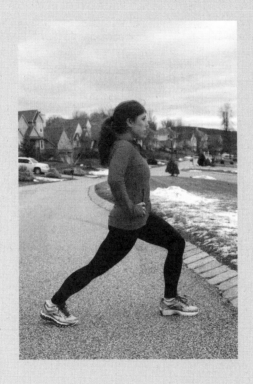

# In this part . . .

- ✔ Find out what's involved in getting started with your walking routine.

- ✔ Select the more appropriate walking type for your weight-loss and health goals and determine how to best implement your walking plan.

- ✔ Learn the ins and outs of available walking equipment and what options may be best for you to help you maximize your results.

- ✔ Discover the correct walking techniques to maximize your results while preventing against injury.

- ✔ Fuel your body to increase weight loss while helping to build strength and endurance.

# Chapter 4

# Hitting the Road

$I$t's time to hit the road and get moving! Whether you are walking to shed pounds, burn belly fat, improve health, or just feel better (or all of the above), you won't start seeing results until you put your foot to the pavement and get started.

As you plan your walking routine, there are many factors you want to consider to make your fitness regimen as easy to stick with as possible. Consider how and where you would enjoy walking the most. Look at the most realistic locations for walking most days. Consider the climate where you live and how the weather will impact your walking workout. And with each of these considerations, keep the goals you hope to achieve with walking in the front of your mind. For instance, if you are walking to reduce stress, planning to walk in a location that can be challenging to get to each day may add to your stress levels rather than decrease them.

Throughout this chapter, I show you the main considerations you want to take into account as you map out your walking routine. I also help you determine the best locations for your workout based on your goals. And, of course, I show you how to be safe, protect yourself against injury, and enhance your compliance with your exercise routine. All it takes is a small amount of planning!

# Deciding Where to Walk

Walking is really one of the easiest exercises you can do because you can do it almost anywhere with little to no equipment (all you need is a good set of footwear to get started).

But even though walking can be done virtually anywhere, it may be challenging to determine where the best locations for your own walking routine may be. When it comes to selecting how and where you will walk, ask yourself these questions:

- ✔ Do you prefer to walk indoors or outdoors?
- ✔ Do you prefer to walk alone or with others (either walking together with friends or family or just walking in the presence of people)?
- ✔ Do you plan to take structured walks for a set time or distance, or just increase your overall daily movement?
- ✔ Will you be motivated on your own to stick with a walking routine, or do you tend to need outside motivation?
- ✔ Do you want to walk near your home or work, or do you prefer to travel to your walking location?

After you answer these questions honestly, you can start to get a sense of your walking personality. You may want to walk with others to prevent a sense of isolation with exercise and to make walking more fun. You may find you need to go to a location to walk rather than walk near your home to ensure compliance. You may determine that you would prefer to walk inside versus outside.

No preference is right or wrong. There isn't a "correct" way to plan a walk. What matters is that you plan a walking routine that will be fun for you. The more you enjoy your walking routine, the easier it will be to stick with it. And compliance with your routine is key to seeing results.

## Discovering walking locations all around you

Even though every walking location can have a downside, one of the great things about walking is that you typically have more than one location available to you to walk. You may not see it now, but there are walking locations all around you if you just know where to look.

### Walking in your own home

You don't even have to go out your own front door to find areas to walk. (See the later section "How and where to walk indoors" for more tips.) You can walk without leaving home with the following strategies:

✔ **Walk the halls:** Walk around the interior of your home by making a path from the living room to the bedroom to the kitchen and back again. You can even walk this path during commercial breaks while watching TV or while talking on the phone to increase your steps.

✔ **Walk the stairs:** Stairs are a great way to increase the intensity and the incline of your walking workout. As you walk up the stairs, you are challenging all the major muscles in your lower body while elevating your heart rate, helping to burn more calories and fat.

✔ **Walk the exterior of your home:** If you love walking outdoors but don't have access to a sidewalk or a safe street to walk on, try walking around the exterior of your house. This tactic allows you to enjoy fresh air while still racking up extra steps

✔ **Utilize walking equipment:** If you have exercise equipment such as a treadmill in your home, this can be a great place to walk. A treadmill allows you to adjust the speed and the incline of your walking workout, allowing you to make it as easy or as challenging as you like.

✔ **Use your DVD player:** Walking DVDs are available to help you increase your steps and burn calories without needing more than a few feet of room. This is a great way to boost your daily steps and fit in a walk in a tight space.

### Walking at work

Every workplace offers the opportunity to increase your daily steps if you just know where to look:

✔ Take the stairs instead of the elevator to increase your steps.

✔ On a break, walk the interior or exterior of your office building.

✔ If your company has an onsite fitness center, see whether you can take a brisk walk on a treadmill before or after your workday.

✔ Talk to coworkers about forming a walking group to encourage regular walking and to make short, brisk walks at work more fun.

✔ Park farther away and walk the length of the parking lot before coming into your building.

### Walking outdoors

The possibilities are limitless when it comes to walking outside (see the later section "The best locations for outdoor walking" for more advice):

✔ Take a stroll down the street in your neighborhood for a relaxing walk.

✔ If possible, walk to nearby stores such as the grocery store instead of driving to fit in more daily steps.

- ✔ Window shop local stores to enjoy the sites while increasing your steps.

- ✔ Power walk at the park or at the local school track to help increase your fitness level and the intensity of your workout.

- ✔ Grab a friend and go for a hike. It's a great way to not only enjoy the outdoors, but to increase the intensity of your walking workout as well.

### Walking while traveling

No matter where you are, there's always the opportunity to find a space to walk. Consider these options:

- ✔ At the airport, take a brisk walk through the terminal while waiting for your flight.

- ✔ When taking a road trip, get out and stretch your legs and aim to briskly walk 500 steps before getting back in the car during rest stops.

- ✔ When out and about — whether you are grocery shopping, at the mall, or enjoying a day with friend — use little tricks such as parking in the last parking spot, taking the stairs instead of the escalator, or taking the long way to the checkout register to help you increase steps and torch calories.

## Finding the best locations based on your goals

Depending on the reason you have decided to start walking, you may find certain locations are better suited to help you reach your goals.

All walking locations offer benefits to your health and well-being. But they all also have their negatives as well. Walking on a high-tech treadmill at the gym can allow for many variants in speed and incline; however, there's a higher cost associated with becoming a gym member. Walking outside to reduce stress can be very relaxing; however, a cold winter or a bad weather day may make walking more difficult. When it comes to finding the best spot for you to walk, you have to weigh the pros versus the cons. The most important factor when you locate the best walking spot for you is how realistic it is that you will walk there on a regular basis. If the location you pick is not convenient, you'll most likely find reasons not to walk, especially on days when you are tired or busy. So make it easy on yourself. Pick the location that's the most convenient for you so you can stick to your routine and reach your goals.

Choosing the wrong location may result in difficulty reaching your goals. For instance, if you want to maximize your ability to shed pounds and inches, choosing a walking location that doesn't allow you to change the intensity of your workout over time may stifle your progress.

The following sections take a look at some of the most common goals and the best locations to achieve them.

### Best location when walking for weight loss

When aiming to lose weight, you want to keep two things in mind: You want to move more throughout the day, and you want to challenge your muscles and your cardiovascular system. Increasing your daily movement during the day is easy. You can track your steps with a pedometer and fit in extra steps with every task you perform.

However, to challenge your muscles and maximize the amount of fat and calories you burn each day, you need to make sure you select a location conducive to this. This involves selecting a walking location that allows you to switch up your workouts. When walking for weight loss, you want to be able to increase your speed and intensity over time. Locations that allow for this include the following:

- Locations with no obstacles that cause you to stop or interrupt your walk (crosswalks, traffic lights, and so on) so you can carry on at a constant speed

- Locations that allow you to vary your terrain by increasing the incline, such as hilly roads or a treadmill with an incline function

- Locations that allow you to incorporate resistance to your workout, such as pushing a stroller or carrying weights

Although the preceding criteria may seem to eliminate many locations, you can actually find locations that incorporate these characteristics almost anywhere. For instance, if you want to walk indoors and walk the interior of your local shopping mall, you can change up the terrain by walking up and down the stairs as part of your walking workout. If you live in a busy city and it's almost impossible to walk without hitting a large number of crosswalks and traffic lights, you can march in place while waiting to cross the road to keep up the intensity of your workout.

### Best locations for fitness walking

If your goal for starting a walking routine is to improve your health, increase your endurance, and build strength, the following criteria are key when selecting your walking location:

- **To increase endurance,** you need to walk for a set duration of time and increase the length of your walk, as well as your speed, over time. Walking on the sidewalk around town, walking on the treadmill, or even walking at the local track all allow you to increase your distance by either walking farther or repeating your walking route (as in walking on a track).

✔ **To build strength,** you need to challenge your muscles while you walk. You can do this in a number of ways, including walking at an incline up a hill or on a treadmill, or walking with resistance, such as wearing weights while walking. Whether you walk uphill, upstairs, or on an incline on the treadmill (or even on a flat surface outside with resistance), you can meet this challenge almost anywhere.

### Best locations for leisure and stress-reducing walking

Perhaps you have taken up walking with the goal of clearing your head and relaxing more. Reducing stress can not only provide you with health benefits, such as lowering blood pressure, but can also help you shed pounds and belly fat.

The key to walking for stress reduction is to select a location that doesn't add to your stress. If you are rushing through rush-hour traffic to get to the gym before coming home to your family, the act of walking may be compounding your stress rather than reducing it. Similarly, if walking at work leads to you having five extra piles of paperwork on your desk by the time you are done, the stress relief you feel while walking will surely come piling back on as soon as you're done.

The key to walking off the stress is to pick a time and location for your walk that won't add to your stress level:

✔ Make sure you enjoy the location you walk in. A scenic park may help to alleviate more stress than walking along a busy street with constant horn-beeping.

✔ Select a time to walk that doesn't compound your stress. If you have a busy job and walking on a lunch break leads to more work and stress, that's not the right time for you to walk. Perhaps instead, you can get to work a few minutes early and walk before you start your day. If you plan to walk with your family but they tend to complain during the walk or want to go back home, that can make your walk less peaceful as well. In this situation, you may want to find a time when you can walk alone to have some peace and quiet as you walk away your stress.

✔ The best choice for stress-reducing walking is a quiet, calming environment. This may be at home, at the gym on a treadmill while you listen to your favorite music, outside as you take in the sights, or even through a shopping mall as you window shop and walk.

Just the act of walking can reduce stress; however, make sure where and how you walk don't add to your daily stress levels.

# Taking Your Walk Outdoors

If you love to be outside, you're in luck. Walking is the perfect outdoor exercise. No matter what the weather, the temperature, or the terrain is like where you live, most of the time, you can get outside and enjoy a walk. Walking outdoors is a great way to boost your energy and reduce your stress levels. Exposure to sunlight has been shown to boost mood. In addition, being in the sun is a great way to increase your vitamin D levels, which have been found in research to help boost mood and fight obesity.

When it comes to walking outdoors, there are really no limitations. You can choose to walk on flat ground, downhill, uphill, rocky terrain, or anything in between. You can walk slowly and take in your surroundings, or you may choose to power walk down the road, working out with your family to talk about your day, or a combination of any of these. Walking outdoors can also be done as a sport. For instance, you may choose to hike outdoors or sign up for a walking event such as a 5k, 10k, or even a half marathon. No matter what your personality is, your fitness goals are, or how much weight you have to lose, walking outside offers a little something for everyone.

## The best locations for outdoor walking

There are almost a countless number of locations you may choose to walk outdoors. You can walk on the beach while feeling the sand between your toes; you can walk through wooded trails as you hike to the top of a mountain; you can walk through the streets of your town or take a stroll at the local park. There's no right or wrong location for walking, especially when walking outdoors. What matters is that you pick the right location for you.

When it comes to picking your outdoor walking location, consider the following:

- ✔ What are your top walking goals?
- ✔ Do you have any walking restrictions, such as a chronic injury?
- ✔ What are your favorite outdoor locations?

Your answers to these questions will help you to narrow down the most appropriate walking locations for you. For instance, if you have chronic knee pain, you would most likely do best walking on a flat surface and avoiding an outdoor walking location with a large number of hills.

If you are at risk for falls or have osteoporosis, avoid any locations with uneven terrain that can increase your risk for falls and fractures. If you're looking to burn the most fat possible during your workout, you want to pick a location that allows you to adjust the intensity of your walk, such as one that allows you to add an incline to your walk.

In addition to deciding on a location that prevents aggravating any injuries and matches your walking goals, you want to decide on a location you enjoy. If you decide to hike through the woods to add hills to your walk but you hate dirt and bugs, you'll most likely have a hard time talking yourself into walking each day. However, if you love looking at the water, walking on the beach each day is something you can look forward to. Also consider the convenience of the location you select for your walk. If you can walk right out your front door and start your walking workout, you're more likely to stick with your workout on a consistent basis than you are if you have to get in the car and drive 20 minutes to reach the beach or the park. Taking all of these factors into account can help you select the perfect location for your personality and goals.

## Outdoor walking considerations

When you choose to walk outdoors, you open yourself up to more variables than if you were to walk indoors, say, on a treadmill. Conditions can change day to day with outdoor walking, which is part of the fun! One day may be chilly and the next day warm. One day the sun may shine brightly whereas the next day you may get hammered by rain.

If you decide to walk outdoors on a regular basis, consider the factors that will vary from day to day so you can be prepared and won't have to skip a workout.

The following sections highlight some important considerations for you to take into account.

### The terrain

A paved road, a quiet sidewalk, or a dirt path are all options when walking outdoors; however, each has its benefits and challenges. Sidewalks can be uneven at times, which can increase the risk of tripping and falling. A paved road allows for street traffic from cars, bikes, and motorcycles, requiring you to obey traffic laws and pay attention to where you are walking to avoid any collisions. Dirt paths often wind through grassy or wooded areas. Trails such as these can help to absorb the impact of your foot striking the ground, placing less pressure on your knees and feet. However, uneven terrain and even puddles from rainwater can increase the risk of falls. Wherever you walk, make sure to pay attention to your surroundings and keep an eye on the road ahead.

### Your safety

You are walking to improve your health and to lose weight; however, if you're not cautious during your walking workout, you may increase your risk of injury or even harm your health. Before heading outdoors on a walk, plan your route. Make sure you know where you are headed and how to get there and get back. Tell a friend or family member where and when you are walking in case they need to reach you. If you'll be walking in an isolated area, make sure to bring your cellphone with you in case of an emergency.

When walking outdoors, coming into contact with animals, extreme weather, and even strangers are all possibilities. It's always best to expect the best but plan for the worst. Walking sticks, noisemakers, and cellphones are all great tools if you find yourself needing to scare off an animal, call for directions or help, or even to keep your balance if you're walking on uneven terrain. Depending on the time of day you choose to walk, keep in mind that you want to be visible, especially if you're walking in a high traffic area. Wear bright colors and reflective apparel when it's dark outside. Make sure to walk on the sidewalk or the shoulder of the road and, most of all, always stay alert.

# Temperature and your walking routine

If you stick with an outdoor walking workout over a period of months, you'll no doubt come into contact with many shifts in temperature and weather patterns. At times, extreme weather like thunderstorms, damaging winds, or very high or very low temperatures may keep you indoors.

There's nothing wrong with switching up your workout on extreme weather days and staying inside instead. However, if you want to be outdoors as often as possible, planning ahead can ensure you can walk safety outside. Before you head outdoors, look at the weather. If it's an extremely hot or cold day, you need to make sure your apparel is appropriate and take precautions such as wearing sunblock, bringing extra water on hot days, or covering your extremities on very cold days. Walking in the rain can be fine; however, rain can increase the risk of slick walking surfaces, so make sure to wear appropriate footwear. If you walk on open roads, you may want to consider bringing your walking workout inside on low visibility days to avoid the possibility of a driver not being able to see you walking on the shoulder of the road.

If you hope to walk outside year-round, make sure to stock up on both cool and hot weather walking essentials, which I outline later in this chapter. In addition, make sure to have a walking backup plan. Even if you are entirely prepared for walking at any temperature, in weather situations such as lightening, hail, or even very low visibility, you should avoid venturing outdoors until the weather has improved. Or you can simply take your walking workout indoors on bad weather days.

### Accounting for cool weather during your walking workout

No matter how motivated you may be to walk and to lose weight, cold weather can be discouraging. But that doesn't mean a dip in the thermometer should put an end to your workout.

Almost everyone can exercise safely in cold weather; however, if you have respiratory conditions such as asthma or chronic obstructive pulmonary disease (COPD), have a heart condition, or suffer from Raynaud's disease, it's best to consult your physician before venturing outdoors. These conditions may require you to take special precautions to ensure you stay safe.

Before heading out, check the weather forecast. Don't just look at the temperature, but also pay attention to the wind chill, any expected precipitation, and the length of time you plan to be outside, as all of these factors play a role in having a safe cold-weather workout.

For instance, if the wind is extreme, even if you dress warmly you may be at an increased risk for frostbite thanks to the wind penetrating your clothes and removing the warm air that can surround your body and insulate it. Or if the forecast calls for rain or snow, wearing waterproof clothing is essential, as you become more vulnerable to the cold when you are wet.

Pay attention to your body and listen to what it tells you when exercising in cold weather. If you begin to feel too cold, your skin starts to feel chapped or irritated, or you feel as though you are having difficultly breathing correctly due to the cold, head indoors. Always make sure to let someone know that you're heading outside to walk, where you are walking, and when you plan to be back, so that person can be on the lookout for you in case something does go wrong along the way.

### Taking cool weather precautions

When walking in cool weather, you need to be extra careful to take care of your body and your skin.

Frostbite is a major concern when the temperature drops, but sunburn and even dehydration can occur in cold weather workouts as well. Taking a few simple precautions can ensure a healthy and happy cool weather workout.

> ✔ **Be on the lookout for signs of frostbite.** When your skin is exposed to freezing temperatures, you can get what is known as frostbite. It most commonly occurs on exposed body parts such as hands and feet, cheeks, nose, and ears. If you begin to experience a stinging sensation, numbness, or a loss of feeling in your skin while out in the cold, you are feeling an early warning sign of frostbite. When you suspect frostbite, go inside out of the cold immediately and slowly warm up the affected area. However, use caution as you warm the area not to rub it, which

can increase damage to your skin. If slowly rewarming your skin doesn't bring back feeling and your skin continues to be numb, seek medical attention right away.

✔ **Know the signs of hypothermia.** When your body temperature dips too low, you suffer from what's known as *hypothermia*. This condition is brought on by the body being unable to produce heat as quickly as it loses it in cold temperatures. When you exercise in extreme cold, wet weather, or high winds, your risk for hypothermia increases. Signs and symptoms of this condition include fatigue, loss of coordination, intense shivering, and slurred speech. This can be a very serious condition, and emergency medical treatment should be sought immediately if hypothermia is suspected.

✔ **Stay well hydrated.** In cool weather, you may not think about increasing your water intake while exercising as you would during a hot weather workout. But no matter what temperature you exercise in, your body still loses fluids through sweat. In fact, the drying power of winter winds can even increase water loss from your skin. Failing to replace this fluid can increase your risk of dehydration. Make sure to drink plenty of fluids before, during, and after your walking workout to maintain adequate hydration. See Chapter 7 for specific hydration guidelines and tips.

✔ **Dress in layers.** The idea of overheating in cold weather may sound funny, but it actually can occur. Many people dress too warmly for a winter workout, forgetting that exercise generates a large amount of heat. The heat generated with exercise can make it feel warmer than it really is. Pair this with excessively warm clothing, and you may feel like you are walking in a sauna. To prevent this, focus on dressing in layers. As you begin to sweat, you can remove layers, and then as your body becomes chilled as sweat evaporates, you can put layers back on.

✔ **Protect your skin from the sun.** Sure, you aren't walking in the hot summer sun, but you can still get sunburned if you aren't careful. In fact, if you walk in snow or at high elevations, you're even more susceptible to sunburn in the winter than in the summer. Before venturing outdoors, make sure to put on a sunblock that blocks both UVA and UVB rays on any exposed skin. Don't forget your lips, either. Cover them with a lip balm that contains sunscreen and wear sunglasses to protect your eyes against the glare from snow and ice.

### Adjusting your workout in hot weather

As the weather warms up and the sun shines down, you may be more motivated to get outdoors and walk. Walking in warmer weather can be a great way to stay active, but as the weather heats up, your workout can be impacted.

Exercising in elevated temperatures can place an increased amount of stress on your body. The combination of the air temperature along with exercise itself elevates your body's core temperature. If your body's temperature rises too high, you can experience serious health conditions. As your temperature rises, your body sends more blood to circulate through your skin to help cool you. However, when this occurs, less blood is available to your muscles, and your heart rate starts to increase. Humid weather, which often comes hand in hand with hot weather conditions, can increase the risk of an excessive rise in your body's core temperature. When humidity is high, sweat doesn't evaporate from your skin as quickly. Sweat evaporation is your body's main way of cooling itself. When this is impaired, your temperature can rise even higher.

However, just because the weather is warming up doesn't mean you have to stop walking outdoors. Taking precautions for warm weather workouts and listening to your body are key to safely walking in warmer conditions. Knowing the signs and symptoms of overheating, making sure you stay hydrated, and dressing appropriately all help to make your walking workout a safe one.

### Taking hot weather precautions

When you are exposed to high temperatures and/or high humidity for long periods of time or you sweat too long without taking in enough fluids, your body's normal cooling system can start to fail. This failure to cool can result in heat-related illnesses, which can range from mild to deadly if left untreated. Everything from painful muscle cramps to lightheadedness and fainting to *heatstroke* (a life-threatening condition where your body temperature rises to greater than 104 degrees Fahrenheit and requires immediate medical treatment) can all result when exercising in hot conditions.

Understanding the precautions to take when exercising in warm weather as well as the signs, symptoms, and treatments for heat-related illness can help keep you safe and healthy when walking in warmer climates.

- ✔ **Know the temperature.** Before heading outdoors to walk, make sure to look at the weather forecast for the day. Know what times of day the temperature is expected to peak as well as the humidity level. Aim to walk at the time of day when the temperature is at the coolest or the humidity level drops.

- ✔ **Know your abilities and fitness level.** If you are new to exercise or walking, your body's tolerance to high heat may be lower than that of a seasoned exerciser. Know your limits and be realistic about your expectations. On high heat days, you may want to plan to take two shorter walks versus one long walk. You may also want to dial down the intensity of your workouts on very hot days and allow your body time to adjust.

✔ **Watch the time you work out.** When walking outside, midday walking tends to be the time of the highest temperatures and increased sun exposure. If you can, plan to walk early in the morning or later in the evening when the temperature drops. If that isn't possible, try moving your walk to a shaded area or performing a lower intensity walking workout during times of very high midday heat.

✔ **Dress appropriately.** Choose clothing that wicks away moisture, helping sweat to evaporate and keeping you cooler. Dark colors tend to absorb more heat from the sun, so choose lighter colored clothing when possible.

✔ **Stay hydrated.** One of the major culprits of heat-related illness is dehydration. Without enough fluids, your body may not be able to sweat enough to cool you properly, causing your core temperature to rise. On average, you want to drink an additional 8 ounces of fluid for every half hour of exercise. However, on very hot or humid days, this amount increases. Drink at least 8 ounces every 15 minutes on these days and don't wait to feel thirsty before you drink. You may also want to consider an electrolyte-rich beverage such as a sports drink on hot days when you find yourself sweating excessively.

✔ **Wear sunscreen.** Summer sun can increase your risk of sunburn. Excessive sun exposure can also increase your risk of skin cancer (as well as premature aging of the skin). Cover exposed body parts with sunblock that blocks both UVA and UVB rays for the best protection. Don't forget to protect your eyes and lips as well: Wear sunglasses that block out glare and damaging sunrays, and cover your lips with a balm that contains sunblock.

✔ **Know the signs and symptoms of heat-related illness.** Heat-related illnesses can become serious quickly. Become familiar with the signs and symptoms and if you experience any, get yourself out of the heat into a cool, dry environment and drink plenty of fluids. If you're not feeling better in 30 minutes, consult your physician for further instructions or seek emergency medical care if your physician is not immediately available. The most common signs and symptoms include the following:

- Muscle cramps

- Headache

- Weakness and fatigue

- Nausea and vomiting

- Excessive sweating

- Dizziness, lightheadedness, and/or fainting

- Low blood pressure

- Rapid heart rate

- Confusion

- Vision problems

On hot weather days, always have a backup plan. If it's too hot or humid to comfortably walk outdoors, consider taking your workout inside. You can go to a gym and walk on a treadmill, walk around the interior of your office building, take a walk inside the local shopping mall, or even just track and increase your steps by using a pedometer daily.

# Walking Indoors

Walking indoors can provide all the same benefits as an outdoor workout. And it has advantages over an outdoor workout as well. When walking indoors, the following apply:

- You don't need to be concerned about whether the weather outside is too hot or cold.

- You don't need to worry about external factors such as avoiding traffic, bugs, or sun exposure, or encountering wild animals.

- You can wear your favorite workout outfit without worrying about dressing in layers, covering yourself in sunblock, or whether the color of your outfit will absorb more heat.

- An indoor walking workout typically has fewer variables, meaning you can be more consistent with your workout duration and intensity.

If an indoor walking workout seems like the type of workout you would enjoy, you just need to determine how you will go about walking indoors so you can best achieve your walking goals. When walking indoors, finding ways to mix up your workout can be a bit more challenging. For instance, varying the intensity of your workout indoors can be a little more difficult as opposed to outdoors, where the landscape can work in your favor, but it can be done. With a little creativity, your walking workout can be just as great as, if not better than, an outdoor walking workout.

## How and where to walk indoors

It may seem like there are more locations to walk outdoors than indoors, but really, you can pretty much walk anywhere anytime. An indoor location is an opportunity to walk. You can walk around the grocery store, an indoor flea market, an indoor track, and the list goes on and on. Where and how you choose to walk are entirely up to you.

When you choose to walk inside, you do want to consider your walking goals. If you plan to walk to shed pounds by focusing on just increasing your daily movement and tracking your steps each day, you can walk almost anywhere.

If you want to speed your results and burn the most fat and calories during your walking workout, you want to have the ability to alter the intensity of your workout by changing your speed, your incline, or resistance. Walking to maximize weight loss and fat loss can require a bit of equipment or creativity when done inside.

### Changing your incline indoors

To help increase the intensity of your walking workout, adding an incline can help you challenge your muscles and burn more fat and calories. Outdoors, this is as easy as walking up a hill, but indoors it can require a bit more creativity. If you walk on a treadmill at your home or a gym that allows you to adjust the incline level, that's all you need to add intensity to your workout. However, if you're walking around your home, a mall, or an office, adding an incline can be a bit more challenging. Using stairs to add an incline to your workout is your best bet. If you are mall walking, after every lap around the mall you can go up the stairs to the next mall level and repeat. You can do the same thing in your home or office by walking a set number of flights of stairs every few minutes during your walking routine. If you don't have access to stairs or are walking in place (such as walking in front of the TV), you can simply march in place, raising your knees higher than you would on a regular walking step, for a set duration of time to pick up the intensity and replicate walking on an incline.

### Changing your resistance indoors

You can add resistance to your walking workout by adding light ankle or hand weights. Whether you walk in your home or in a public area like a mall, you can bring your weights with you to use during your walk. Some people find that performing more resistance exercises while walking — such as doing shoulder presses with light weights while walking or adding lunges to a walk — is easier to do at home than outdoors where they're concerned with uneven terrain or even the idea of others looking at them while they're exercising.

### Changing your speed indoors

If you have access to a treadmill, adjusting your speed can be quick and easy. If you're walking in a limited space, adjusting your speed can pose more of a challenge. For instance, if you walk around your living room, do you have space to power walk? Probably not. However, you can still push yourself to cover more steps in a shorter amount of time to increase your speed. You can also look for opportunities in larger spaces, such as shopping centers, to walk quickly in straight open areas and then slow down in more crowded spaces to add interval training to your workout.

# Indoor walking considerations

When it comes to walking indoors, consider the following factors to make sure you can safely and effectively complete the walking workout you want to achieve your desired goals:

- ✔ **Space:** When walking indoors, you must take space into consideration. Unlike walking outdoors where you have access to as much open space as you could possibly desire, indoor walking can be a bit more limiting. When walking indoors, you take into account that you'll most likely need to repeat your desired route over and over.

- ✔ **Equipment:** You can use as little or as much equipment as you like when walking inside. If increasing speed, distance, and intensity are part of your walking goals, finding a way to access a treadmill either by purchasing one or going to a gym that has one can be a great asset to your workout. A treadmill allows you to easily adjust your speed and incline level over and over again without having to find access to stairs or ramps, or having to march in place. A pedometer is also a fantastic piece of equipment to consider using when walking indoors. It allows you to track your overall steps so you can see just how much and how far you have walked every day.

- ✔ **Accessibility:** When choosing to walk indoors, make sure you have access to where you want to walk on a regular basis. If you walk in your home, accessibility is easy to come by. However, if you walk at a shopping center, you need to be able to drive to the shopping center and can only walk when it is open. If you walk inside your office building, you need to find alternatives on days you're not working, such as weekends, if your building isn't open.

- ✔ **Safety:** Although walking outdoors can increase the need to take safety precautions such as battling changing weather conditions or uneven terrain, walking indoors can have safety risks as well. If you choose to walk on a treadmill, make sure you know how to operate the emergency shutoff switch if you need to stop walking at once. If you plan to walk up and down stairs, make sure you have access to a handrail in case you lose your balance. And just as when walking outdoors, if you plan to walk inside a public location, such as a shopping center, make sure you let someone know where you're going and when you expect to be back in case of any emergencies.

# Chapter 5

# Walking Workout Equipment and Preparation

*A*s you plan your walking workout, you're most likely deciding on a few factors. Will you walk outdoors or indoors? What time of day do you plan to walk? Will your walks be fast-paced fitness walks or more casual strolls? As you determine the answers to these questions, you may think about ways to make your walk easier or more effective. For instance, if you plan to walk outdoors, what can you use to protect yourself against harsh weather or to help stabilize yourself on uneven terrain? If you walk indoors, what equipment is best to enhance your walk? If you are focused on generally increasing your overall daily physical activity, what are the best tools for tracking this and helping you to be more active overall?

Although when it comes to walking all you really need is a pair of supportive footwear and a place to walk, additional equipment can help to make your walk more effective, safer, and even more comfortable. You may already be aware of some of the walking products and equipment on the market, such as treadmills and walking shoes, but other equipment you may not have heard of. Throughout this chapter, I introduce you to the many walking products available, what they do, and how they may be of use to you.

Because determining the best equipment for you, such as the best footwear, can be overwhelming at times, I also give you guidelines on how to select the best equipment and what may or may not be appropriate for you based on your weight loss and health goals. Although there's no need to buy all, or any, of this equipment to walk away the pounds, you may find some of these products help you to see results more quickly and even make your workout more fun in the process.

# How Walking Equipment Can Impact Your Workout

Can you walk without fancy equipment? Absolutely! However, it may benefit you to consider some of the new technology available and how it may enhance your workout. Technology has come a long way across many categories, including fabrics, electronics, equipment, apps, wearable technology, websites, and even at-home healthcare. Within each category are many fascinating and very useful products that can help you assess your current health and weight and track changes and improvement in your overall health and fitness levels. In addition, some of these options may help to prevent or reduce pain from injuries, allow you to walk safely in varying terrains and weather conditions, and make your walk more fun and enjoyable overall.

As you go through this chapter, I introduce you to many options; however, because fitness equipment and technology are constantly changing and expanding, I provide additional information, such as product comparison buying guides and stores (big box retailers and hard-to-find specialty stores) that sell these products (and coupons), on my website at www.erinpalinski-author.com. As you'll see as you discover more about the various products available to you, some may come in quite handy as you get started with a walking program or look to maximize your workout to speed your results. Not every product is appropriate or necessary for everyone, but increasing your knowledge about what is available in the marketplace can only help to improve your overall fitness and weight-loss results.

## Why equipment is essential to your workout

When it comes to walking off the weight, all you really need is to wear supportive footwear and put one foot in front of the other. However, depending on your health, your age, when you walk, where you walk, and how often you walk, certain products and equipment can help to reduce your risk of injury and therefore prevent you from becoming sidelined from your walking workout. For instance, with the proper footwear, foot care, posture, and stretching, many of the most common walking injuries can be prevented. If you can only afford one walking product, I recommend choosing a quality walking shoe. A good shoe can help to prevent pain, discomfort, and injury in the foot, knee, hip and even back.

### Finding the right fit

Fit is always the number one factor when it comes to selecting your footwear, and it should come before all other considerations, including technology, reviews, or fashion. A proper fit keeps you from developing ingrown toenails, blisters, and irritation. When it comes to defining a properly fitting shoe, footwear should be snug everywhere, tight nowhere, and provide enough room for you to wiggle your toes. Other criteria and footwear and foot care buying guides are listed on my website. I also recommend certain shoes, such as Reebok, and foot care that you can find at big retailers like Sears as well as specialty stores like Best Insoles (www.bestinsoles.com) and Amazing Socks (www.amazingsocks.com).

### Maintaining correct posture

Posture is essential when it comes to preventing injuries. Proper posture not only reduces slip-and-fall injuries, but it also strengthens your core to prevent and manage injuries. When walking, remember to keep your shoulders down and back, while gently pulling your abdominal muscles in. Chapter 6 provides specific details and guidelines for the right posture to maintain when walking. If you forget posture often, you can wear full body braces or straps that keep your shoulders back or try a lower back support elastic wrap. Walgreens and specialty stores like The Brace Shop (www.braceshop.com) or CWI Medical (www.cwimedical.com) have a wide selection.

### Preparing your muscles

To make sure you can stay on track with your walking workout and avoid stiff muscles and discomfort, it's important to care for your muscles before and after each workout through stretching, massage, and hot or cold therapy as needed. Chapter 6 provides a list of the best stretching exercises along with proper warm-up and cool-down strategies.

When stretching, having an exercise mat that is easy to carry and store can be quite helpful. You can find a large selection at retailers such as wayfair.com. In addition, finds such as TriggerPoint (www.tptherapy.com) and Moji (www.gomoji.com) that have great high-tech, high-fashion products for feet and foam rollers and massage balls can be quite helpful. If you have an actual injury, and your physician has cleared you for walking, you can find appropriate braces, wraps, and ointments at retailers such as Walgreens. You can also find these options and more at medical stores like The Brace Shop.

However, any time you have discomfort, pain, or an injury, make sure to see your healthcare provider first and always follow his recommendation for treatment. Don't self-diagnose or self-treat an injury.

## Getting the best equipment to stay safe and comfortable

Depending on how you walk, where you walk, and your walking goals, your equipment needs may vary. For example, say you mostly walk outdoors after work. In the fall, after the time change, when it starts to get dark early, you may have safety concerns about continuing to walk in the dark. You can continue to walk outdoors even after the sun goes down, but having the right equipment is essential to staying safe.

For starters, you want to wear reflectors if you're walking near cars so you'll be seen. No need to get nervous thinking you have to wear a big, bulky reflector jacket, because now you can actually have fun with stick-on reflectors, like Lightweights for Clothing and Gear Power Reflectors, or a glow stick with a whistle; you can find both at REI (www.rei.com). If you bring your dog, be sure to have a dog leash with a reflector, which can be found at retailers such as Petsmart. Wearing a headlamp can also be a great way to enhance your vision and help you avoid potholes or bumps in the terrain that could cause injury. You can find headlamps at Backwoods (www.backwoods.com) or most electronics, sports, or camping stores like Sports Authority.

In addition to when you walk, where you walk, your fitness and health level, your comfort with technology, and even the weather all impact what equipment may be helpful to you. Whatever your needs, here are some things to consider:

- ✔ **Hydration:** Staying hydrated is not only essential for endurance and fitness, but can also help to promote weight loss. To help you drink while you walk, look into options such as BPA-free water bottles, fitness belts with holders for water bottles, or hands-free hydration packs. Check websites like www.salomon.com and www.rei.com for a wide selection.

- ✔ **Walking poles:** If you're looking to build strength and enhance your metabolism, walking poles can help. Choose resistance poles to work your triceps, chest, and shoulders along with your lower body to burn more calories. They're also good for balance and support. I like the walking pole sold by hälsa (www.halsamat.com) for its resistance. The Health Mark Trekking Pole, which you can find at many sporting good stores, big box retailers, and online, is interesting because it contains a built-in pedometer to help track your steps. When purchasing a walking pole, you want to factor in criteria such as carbon versus aluminum and the weight of the pole for the best personal option for you.

- ✔ **Waist-, arm-, or backpacks:** You should be hands-free, but you'll still need to carry the essentials like a water bottle, your keys, sunscreen,

ID, money, and your mobile phone. Space, comfort, budget, and fashion may also be important to you. I like the Ultimate Direction Strider Hydration Pack, which you can get at Kohls and which contains compartments for carrying all your essentials when walking, or other items from specialty stores such as eBags.com.

✔ **Earbuds:** The power of a pumped-up playlist can energize your workout. So, you'll want a pair of earbuds for your phone that fit as snugly as your sneakers, deliver rich sound, and perform well in puddles of ear sweat. The JayBird BlueBuds X, which can be purchased at large retailers such as Best Buy and Amazon.com, offer high quality audio performance and a sweat-proof, secure fit that is ideal for exercise.

✔ **Sun blockers:** If you walk during the day, sunscreen is essential. Block UVA and UVB rays with a pair of sporty sunglasses and sunscreen lotion. Gray lenses block the brightest lights, while red sharpens depth perception, ideal for hiking on shady trails. A small bottle of sunscreen and lip balm with sun protection on a clip are ideal.

✔ **Cold weather:** Don't forget your handwarmers! They now come in packs that manually warm up through chemicals in the pack (see HotHands on drugstore.com), and some are battery operated. If it's snowy and icy, you can buy ice grippers to attach to your shoes. And, don't forget to wear layers because your body will heat up during your walk and you may need to take off a layer.

✔ **Hot weather:** Wear lightweight, light-colored clothing or moisture-wicking materials, such as polypropylene, CoolMaxÂ, and SupplexÂ, that evaporate sweat quickly and cool your skin. Or invest in new sun-protective pieces: More and more companies are creating clothes with an ultraviolet protection factor, or UPF, rating to block harmful UV-rays. Breathable shoes can help as well. Try mesh versus leather (I discuss how to select the best shoe for you later in this chapter).

✔ **Heart rate monitors:** If you have any health condition, walking in extreme temperatures can be taxing on your body and is not recommended. Before heading out on very hot or very cold days, speak to your healthcare provider first. If you are cleared to walk despite the weather, keep an eye on your heart rate. Watching your heart rate with a heart rate monitor is ideal (try Heart Rate Monitors USA at www.heartratemonitorsusa.com).

✔ **Rain:** Don't let the rain stop you! You can find rain ponchos that pack up to the size of a coin purse. For your phone, Topeak and Eddie Bauer have great smartphone dry bags, which are a must. You can even bring a Rite in the Rain notebook (from www.rakuten.com) to jot down your thoughts on a halfway break.

   ✔ **Long walks or hiking:** If you're going on long walks in groups where cell coverage isn't ideal or in case your phone's battery dies, you should bring a walkie-talkie for safety. I like the Motorola Talkabout MS Series that you can find at Best Buy (`www.bestbuy.com`). Less costly ones that are just as good are also available. Alternatively, a portable solar charger is a must to keep your phone charged. A compact first aid kit is also a must, which you can hook to your waist pack or backpack. Use the Key Chain Carabiner Clips you can find at Oriental Trading (`www.orientaltrading.com`) to hook water bottles, sunscreen, compact compasses with thermometers, and other items to your packs. And if you want to capture memories during your walk, a GoPro camera (`www.gopro.com`) can be ideal to capture video to share on social media.

# How to Select the Best Walking Shoes

When it comes to walking for exercise, the single most important piece of equipment that you need is a pair of supportive, well fitting, walking shoes. Without the proper shoes, your risk of injury and discomfort greatly increases, which lessens your chances of staying on track with your walking routine. Although the correct footwear is essential, knowing how to identify the right footwear for you can feel overwhelming.

Depending on where you walk, how often, and the type of walking you do, your footwear needs vary. In addition, if you have any orthopedic issues or health conditions, such as diabetes, your footwear needs may be more specialized. Think about your planned walking routine as well as any preexisting injuries, previous foot discomfort (such as frequent blisters), or health conditions that impact your feet that you may have. Once you have identified how you walk and any specialized needs you may have, you can start to understand what form of footwear is best suited for you.

Fit is key to a great walking shoe. You want to avoid rubbing that can cause blisters or pinching that cuts off circulation. The shoes should be snug, but roomy enough for your toes to wiggle around. And, the shape of your foot (whether you're flat-footed or have high or normal arches) also determines comfort. You'll need to try on several pairs to see the differences, and when you find the one, you'll know. Stores like REI and The Walking Shoe have excellent salespeople to guide you, or you can try on several at home at no cost by shopping online at `www.zappos.com` or `www.macys.com`, which offer free shipping and free returns. I have a list of additional shoe stores that offer round-trip free shipping on my website.

When it comes to walking shoes, remember that they are designed specifically for walking and should only be used for that purpose. Walking requires a shoe providing a low, rounded heel with good support and should be light-weight and allow your foot to breathe.

One of the most important things to look for is a soft landing when walking, to reduce the impact walking has on your bones and joints. However, when looking at the thickness of the sole of your shoe, don't overdo it either. Make sure the shoe still remains flexible, especially at the toe.

Other factors that are also important to consider include technology available with the shoe, fashion, weight, fabrics, and your fitness level (whether you're a power walker or more of a leisurely walker). The use of your shoe matters too. Think about whether you're walking indoors, outdoors, or in particular weather conditions, as well as your health.

## Walking shoes for indoor walking

You may be walking at work, at home, on a treadmill at the gym, on a track at the gym, or even at the mall. When walking indoors, a lightweight shoe that's breathable is typically your best option, because your climate is controlled and you don't have to worry about becoming too warm or too cold. However, depending on the type of walking you're doing, finding a shoe with appropriate support is important.

If you plan to power walk on the treadmill or indoor track, having good support is key. Make sure your shoe contains enough shock resistance to protect your body from the pounding of fast walking. Try out a few shoes and make sure they feel flexible enough to walk in while providing shock absorption and good arch support. Some companies that provide a good selection of indoor walking shoes include Rebok (www.reebok.com/us), Adidas (www.adidas.com/us/), and Sneakers 4 U (www.sneakers4u.com).

## Walking shoes for outdoor walking

When it comes to walking outdoors, the weather conditions and terrain are the biggest factors in selecting appropriate footwear. If you typically walk in a warm climate, look for lightweight, ventilated walking shoes such as those with mesh panels. Mesh is cooler than leather and dries faster when your feet sweat. In addition, try pairing your walking shoe with socks that wick away sweat, to help keep your feet as dry and comfortable as possible. If you walk at a slow pace, you may also look into walking sandals as well for extra breathability.

If you walk in colder weather, aim for a full leather shoe for extra warmth. Looking for an all-terrain sole is also helpful to prevent slips in ice or snow. If you plan to walk in extreme weather conditions or on uneven terrain, crampons, ice grippers, and other terrain sole attachments are quite useful for safety and endurance and can be found at retailers such as Zappos, (www.zappos.com).

## Walking shoes for varying fitness levels

Your current fitness level and walking goals can also help to determine your footwear selection. If your main goal is comfort when walking, a great brand to look for is Ryka Radiant, which was voted most comfortable walking shoe by *Fitness Magazine*. However, for power walkers, this same magazine selected New Balance 615 as the most supportive option.

If you plan to walk more casually at a slower pace or are mostly focusing on increasing your steps, you may find yourself walking barefoot at times (especially if you enjoy walking on the beach). But if you have medical conditions that can impact your circulation, especially those that can impact circulation in your legs and feet, such as diabetes, it's vital to never walk barefoot as this could lead to wounds and infections. However, if you love the feel of walking barefoot, but want more protection, one option to look into is Xero Shoes (www.xeroshoes.com). If you do have any medical or orthopedic condition, make sure to ask your physician first whether these would be appropriate for you.

If your main goal of walking is not only to lose weight but also to increase muscle tone, look into a walking shoe that helps promote increased toning. For instance, the Avia i-Burn has a rocker technology that causes your heel and forefoot to sink and rise as you walk. The manufacturer states that this technology helps you feel as though you're walking at a 5 percent incline on a treadmill. Another toning shoe option is the Reebok EasyTone Grace. This shoe has a bouncy feature, which can make your toning walk seem more fun. And the more fun you have, the more often you will walk!

## Walking shoes for orthopedic problems

If you have flat feet, bunions, plantar fasciitis, or any variety of foot issue, orthopedic shoes can make your walk not only safer, but also more comfortable. In fact, wearing the correct orthopedic shoe can help to prevent, treat, and even reduce pain caused by many foot conditions. It can also help to prevent these conditions from worsening into a chronic, painful condition that may keep you from walking on a regular basis.

Orthopedic shoes have come a long way, and in addition to providing extra comfort and protection, they can be quite stylish too. These shoes typically provide extra depth, shock absorption, and support and come in a variety of shapes and sizes to accommodate any foot size and any form of walking. If you have orthopedic foot conditions, speak to your podiatrist about the best and safest footwear for your specific condition and planned form of exercise.

When selecting an orthopedic shoe, you may want to visit a specialty store whose selection and service cater to your needs, such as www.healthyfeetstore.com. These stores have shoes uniquely designed for orthopedic problems, diabetics, arthritis, bunions, and plantar fasciitis, and they even have shoes for after surgeries as well.

But as always, refer to your healthcare team's advice when it comes to selecting the most appropriate footwear for your needs.

## Walking shoes for health issues

Certain health conditions can put you more at risk for injuries when walking. In addition, other health conditions can impact circulation, leading to poor wound healing. With conditions such as these, it's vital that you practice proper foot care and select the best footwear for your individual needs to cut down on your risk of wounds that can lead to infection.

Individuals with diabetes need to be especially careful when walking. Ill-fitting footwear can increase the risk of blisters and wounds, which, if left untreated, can result in infection and, in extreme cases, amputation. In Chapter 12, I outline the guidelines for foot care with diabetes and discuss the steps you need to take daily to ensure wound prevention and early detection. In addition, with diabetes, it's very important to visit your podiatrist regularly and discuss what footwear would be best for you when walking. With a diagnosis of diabetes, some insurance companies even provide reimbursement for your footwear. However, regardless of whether you purchase your footwear on your own or your insurance company provides it for you, make sure you always discuss your choices with your physician first to get the best option for your individual needs.

Health conditions such as arthritis, osteoporosis, and degenerative joint disease can impact your gait when walking, increasing your risk for falls and injuries. With these conditions, you should speak with your podiatrist and/or physical therapist about specific considerations to keep in mind when selecting your walking shoe. Depending on your needs, you may need a shoe with a thicker sole for extra shock absorption, an extra-flexible shoe to aid in balance, or a shoe with an all-terrain sole to help protect against slip and fall accidents, especially if walking outside. Walking with health conditions is possible, and very often may even help to improve your condition. But safety is always the first priority, so always speak to your physician first to determine what is best for your individual needs.

# How Apparel Can Impact Your Walking Workout

You've probably given a lot of thought to the best footwear for you when walking, but most likely you haven't given other apparel much consideration. You probably just figure as long as you are wearing comfortable clothing when walking, that works just fine. And it can. However, fitness clothing has come a long way in the past decade or two, and choosing the right apparel can aid your workout. Depending on when and wear you walk, the temperature and weather conditions can play a major role in the best clothing and apparel for you. Choosing the right apparel can increase your comfort when walking, allowing you to walk longer and more often, maximizing your workout benefits.

Moisture-wicking fabrics are a great choice for staying dry while sweating, especially if you walk in warm temperatures. However, even in colder weather, these fabrics have benefits. When layering, wear moisture-wicking fabric against your skin, and layer it with other, warmer fabrics to keep out the cold. According to REI.com, natural fibers are superior to synthetic fibers when it comes to keeping you dry. However, whether you choose synthetic or natural fibers, look for certified sports performance moisture wicking and antibacterial properties.

Choosing the right fabrics can make a world of difference in having a comfortable walk. You have many options depending on your needs, including the following:

- A 100 percent opaque cotton fabric is all natural and breathes in warm weather, and the opaqueness ensures you have full coverage.

- Bamboo is another great breathable, all-natural fabric that absorbs moisture quickly.

- Fleece is a great synthetic option for cold-weather walks.

- Merino fabric, which is antibacterial, all-natural wool from sheep, is ultra warm, sweat-wicking, and ethical (biodegradable and sustainable).

- If you are facing winds, especially cold winds, a hard- or soft-shell, waterproof, and windproof outer layer will cut the cold, especially if you're layering with fleece or merino wool underneath.

Weaving techniques and other properties can also make a difference:

- A great construction technique is bonded or seamless technology that uses adhesives rather than seams to bond fabric. It gives you a smooth look and a chafe-free experience.
- Antibacterial and hypoallergenic fabric allows skin to remain odor free.
- Compression garments help improve circulation, which feeds more oxygen to muscles, reduces lactic acid buildup, and reduces muscle fatigue, thereby enhancing performance.

When looking at all the fabrics and options available to you, Sweaty Betty (www.sweatybetty.com) is a great find, offering fun, fashionable designs in a wide array of fabrics.

Fit is also important when choosing the right apparel for your walking workout. Watch out for areas where skin rubs against skin — between your toes, thighs, and under your arms, which can lead to friction and chafing of the skin. To help you feel comfortable under your fitness clothes, performance undergarments can be quite helpful. Aim to choose sweat-wicking fabrics over cotton, which gets wet easily and stays wet, contributing to chafing in sensitive spots.

To help create a barrier to moisture, use a small amount of petroleum jelly or Runner's Lube, a nonstaining cream made from lanolin, zinc oxide, and benzocaine that can be found in many sporting goods or drugstores, such as Eastern Mountain Sports (www.ems.com) or drugstore.com.

Fitness apparel and clothing are constantly evolving. Wearable electronics like headphones and watches have been commonplace among fitness enthusiasts. However, in the past few years, wearable technology has begun to evolve even further to include items such as T-shirts, smart bras, socks, and full body fitness tops and bottoms that have once-wired technology built in. This clothing, provided by companies such as Athos (www.liveathos.com), has sensors and Bluetooth technology that captures electromyography (EMG) muscle activity, heart rate, skin temperature, and breathing, providing you with a vast amount of information about every workout.

## Choosing the right socks

Socks can often go unnoticed, but in addition to the proper footwear, socks are one of the most important pieces of apparel you need for effective and healthy walking. When you walk, pressure points on your feet, moisture buildup from sweat, and the force and impact of each step can lead to blisters. However, socks are your first line of defense against this. If they bunch up, don't fit correctly, or leave your feet moist, your risk of blisters (and need to put walking on hold for a period of time) increases.

Socks that provide moisture-wicking fabric and have light padding in key areas, such as the heel and ball of the foot, can protect your feet from the risk of irritation and blisters, and may even add additional cushioning to each step. Various socks for walking on the market provide these features. One such sock available at retailers such as REI is WrightSock, which is considered a leader in performance socks. Whatever sock you select, look for a few specific features for the greatest benefit:

- ✔ Choose a sock shaped like your foot to allow it to stay in place and prevent bunching. Elastic or ribbing helps to ensure that socks stay put.

- ✔ Look for gender-specific socks, because men and women have differently shaped feet. This allows for a snugger fit.

- ✔ Choose socks made in wicking fabrics to help fight against blisters, such as CoolMax, Dri-Fit, Sorbtek, or SmartWool. Most sport stores, such as www.backcountry.com, carry quality walking socks.

- ✔ If you're a techie, you may love www.sensoriafitness.com. Its socks have built-in textile sensors that act like a personal walking coach. They work with a Bluetooth smart anklet that provides you with information on your walk, such as your speed and steps, and also gives you feedback on your foot landing technique and even weight distribution as you walk, which may help in the fight against injuries.

## *Wearing the right undergarments*

You may not have given much thought to your undergarments before starting your walking program, but if you choose the wrong options, you'll certainly recognize it during your workout.

Choosing the wrong fabric or the wrong fit can lead to discomfort, chafing, and even increased risk of skin infections. Use the same criteria when looking for undergarments that you use when purchasing footwear or outerwear for your workout. Look for options that fit well; are made of breathable, wicking fabrics; and are comfortable.

Although the choices of undergarments are vast, some have been found to outperform the rest. If you want to review your options along with the pros and cons of each, check out my website for a buying guide comparing everything from ASICS to Barely There for women and everything in between to help you make the best selection possible.

If you wear moisture-wicking fabrics, undergarments are not always a necessity, especially if you wear antibacterial fabric like Get Set Go shorts from Under Armour. However, for men, long endurance workouts can cause irritation and chafing. When buying underwear, men should consider anatomical support provided by a full front pouch that provides the benefit of a jockstrap. Check out the Jack Adams Trainer Trunk and other options at The Underwear Expert (www.underwearexpert.com).

When it comes to choosing undergarments for women, steer clear of lace and satin, as these fabrics are less breathable and may cause irritation. If you suffer from bladder leakage, don't let it hold you back from regular exercise. Companies such as Dear Kate (www.dearkates.com) make "leak-free lingerie" athletic options, which can be the perfect fit for helping you feel comfortable and confident as you walk.

Sports bras are also an essential component of the walking woman's wardrobe. Selecting a good-fitting sports bra can minimize the movement of your chest, preventing discomfort when walking. In addition, it can wick moisture away from the skin, allowing for air flow and fighting against chafing. When choosing a sports bra, make sure that the straps don't dig into your shoulders, that the band around your lower chest isn't too tight or too loose, and that the fabric is lightweight and soft. Even if you've had a mastectomy, you can still walk with confidence and comfort. Visit www.healthproductsforyou.com for a great line of post-mastectomy apparel that will have you looking and feeling great while walking.

# Miscellaneous Walking Accessories

No matter where or when you walk, some tools and equipment are almost essential to allowing you to gain the greatest benefit from your walk. As I mention throughout this book, walking really is the most versatile and least expensive form of exercise there is. All you need is a good pair of supportive footwear, and you're set. And that's true. However, having some tools on hand, if they work for your lifestyle and budget, can help to maximize your workout.

If you can make your walk more effective at burning calories and fat each and every minute, you'll see results faster, helping you to stay motivated to reach your long-term goals. You in no way need these tools to be able to achieve your goals; however, they can make the journey to achieving your goals a little easier if they work for you.

## Indoor walking

If you walk inside your home, unless your home is very large, your total walking space may be limited. Even so, you can still increase your overall daily steps by walking back and forth, walking up and down stairs, or even marching in place. However, using a treadmill can add much more versatility to your indoor walk by allowing you to increase your speed, incline, and distance. If you're in the market for a treadmill, do your research ahead of time to see what features are most important to you.

If walking at work is possible, you can certainly fit in brief walks before and after you begin working as well as on any breaks. Walking while you work can really help you to rack up the steps and burn calories. If you have the option, ask for a treadmill desk, or simply stand up when typing or walk in place when possible. The www.trekdesk.com is a great option for higher budgets, and my site has options for those on a tighter budget as well.

## Outdoor walking

If you walk in the city, you may find some unique opportunities as well as challenges when it comes to walking. To help enhance the intensity of your workout, especially if hills are few and far between, look into using a walking pole. One that folds for easy storage is great for city living, like the Black Diamond Ultra Distance sold online at www.backcountry.com and www.ems.com. In heavily congested areas, make sure you take your safety seriously as well. Use reflective gear or clothes and walk against traffic, especially when the sun goes down. And, you may want to add other unique equipment such as Rearview Behind Sunglasses that have a rearview mirror feature (try Dick's Sporting Goods at www.dickssportinggoods.com). As you walk, always be aware of your surroundings, keep your head up, and stay alert. If you plan to use your phone when walking, use Siri on your iPhone combined with earbuds for your phone to talk, text, and listen to music so your hands are free and you can stay alert. If you do need to stop, such as to wait for a light to cross an intersection, keep walking in place to maintain your heart rate.

If you walk outdoors in a rural setting, make sure your footwear has good traction to fight against slips and falls. Shoes with all-terrain soles can help, or you can add Yaktrax Walkers to your shoes, which are ropelike additions to the bottom sole. Many retailers carry them. Crampons are also useful for rough terrain. Depending on the time of year you are walking, you may also want to carry insect repellent. To cut down on the amount of items you need to carry with you, look into using a Hide-A-Key Realistic Rock Outdoor Key Holder, available at retailers like Home Depot, which not only allows you to walk with fewer items, but helps to prevent accidental lock-outs caused by forgetting or losing your keys while walking. And, if you want to make your walk more entertaining, think about using binoculars or a monocular for walks in scenic locations. Or even bring a camera to document memorable walks. The more fun you make your walk, the more likely you are to stick with it!

# Chapter 6

# The Science of Walking

**S**o you're ready to start your walking workout. It's easy — all you have to do is head out the door, place one foot in front of the other, and you're on your way. Simple, right? Not so fast. Yes, it's true that you already know how to walk. You've been doing it since pretty much your first birthday.

However, just because you know how to walk doesn't mean that you always walk correctly. When you start walking for a long duration to increase exercise, it's imperative that you have correct technique. A poor walking technique can do everything from increase muscle soreness to increase your risk of injury, and can even slow your weight-loss results.

But if you take the time to refine your walking technique and make sure you are walking correctly for the entire duration of your walking workout, you'll not only see weight-loss results faster, but you'll improve your overall fitness and posture as well.

Throughout this chapter I show you the correct way to walk (for instance, walking for exercise requires a slightly different technique than just taking a leisurely stroll). I also help you identify correct posture and show you how to determine whether your posture needs work. This chapter also helps you to understand the most common walking-related injuries, what causes them, and how you can prevent them. Finally, I wrap up the chapter with the proper warm-up and cool-down techniques that are vital to incorporate into your walking workout every day. Are you ready to get started?

# What Is Gait?

The term *gait* is defined as a person's manner of walking. An abnormal gait, which can occur due to disease such as arthritis or even from previous injuries such as fractures, can impact your overall ability to walk as well as increase your risk of future injury.

To see how important a correct gait is, give this activity a try: Stand barefoot with your feet a bit wider than hip width apart and roll your feet inward slightly so that you're only using your big toe. Now, take a few steps. Do any muscles seem to be working harder than others? Do you feel some muscles working that you don't typically feel when you walk? If you walked like this for a distance, you would most likely feel a pull in the inside of your knee. And repeated walking this way can cause your knee to become out of alignment, increasing injury risk.

The same issue can happen if you place too much weight on your smallest toe when walking or walk mostly on your heels rather than the ball of the foot. Anytime you walk off balance or don't utilize your entire foot, you cause other muscles in your lower body to be overused, and this can lead to pain and injury, which over time can keep you from walking. That's why a correct gait is so important.

## Correct walking techniques

You know that song "the knee bone's connected to the thigh bone, the thigh bone's connected to the hip bone . . ."? It's true; your bones are all connected as well as tendons, ligaments, and even your muscles.

If you throw a bone, joint, or muscle out of whack, it causes a chain reaction to the bones and joints in the rest of your body. A poor walking technique may not only lead to an increased risk of bunions on your feet but can also increase the risk of knee pain, hip pain, back pain, and so on. If you plan to increase the amount of walking you do on a regular basis to lose weight, it's important that you walk correctly. If you don't, these aches and pains will start to present themselves, which can make continuing with your walking routine a challenge.

Take a look at how to position yourself for the healthiest walk possible:

1. **Start by standing with your feet exactly hipbone width apart, not wider or closer.**

   This stance should allow your legs to be stacked straight up and down from your feet to your hips. Your toes should point forward (every toe from the big toe to the pinky toe should be facing forward — not turned outward or inward). Picture having headlights on your hipbones, knee-caps, and big toes. Make sure all of your headlights are facing straight ahead. This position allows for the least amount of wear and tear on your ankles, knees, hips, and feet.

2. **Now take a step forward, making sure that your foot lands with your heel first.**

   To do this, you must flex your foot at the ankle. If you are unable to do this, examine your footwear first. Overly stiff shoes can impede this motion, which can increase injury risk. Make sure you choose support-ive shoes that also allow flexibility in your feet and ankles.

3. **After your heel hits the ground, roll onto the ball of your foot.**

   The ball of your foot is essentially the midsection of your foot — the part in front of the arch but behind the toes. As the ball of your foot hits the floor, your toes should be flexed. As you roll onto the ball of your foot, pay attention to how you do it. If you roll to one side or the other, prac-tice walking slowly and making sure the entire ball of your foot presses against the floor as you step. If you are able to do this barefooted, but not when wearing shoes, it's possible your shoes are too stiff.

4. **Use your toes — all of them!**

   As you roll through the ball of your foot with your step, you want to roll forward onto your toes. Your pinky toe should be the first to hit the floor while big toe should be the last. All of your toes should come into contact with the ground, in succession. As you continue to walk, the toes should leave the ground in the same order they came in contact with it — pinky toe first, big toe last. Skipping a toe can impair your balance as well as place unneeded stress on the bones and joints in your feet.

How did you do? Does it feel odd to walk this way? If so, just take time prac-ticing this technique over and over.

Walk slowly and really pay attention to how you are walking. It may seem silly, but improving your gait pays off in the long run.

## *Achieving proper posture*

Just as proper gait is vital to keeping your body healthy while walking, pos-ture is equally important. *Posture* is the way in which you hold your body when sitting or standing.

Poor posture can throw your body out of alignment, increasing the risk of everything from falls to injury to even impacting how you breathe. In addition, poor posture looks bad. If you stand up tall and utilize good posture, you automatically look slimmer (even before you drop pounds and inches from walking!).

### Start by standing correctly

So what is correct posture and how can you achieve it? Take a look:

1. **Start by standing up straight while you think of yourself as being tall.**

   Picture a string at the top of your head pulling your hips, chest, and chin upwards.

2. **As you stand up tall, don't arch your back.**

   Keep your back straight and pull your abdominal muscles in. Tuck your bottom in by rotating your hips forward slightly, which helps to prevent arching.

3. **Watch where you look.**

   You don't want to be leaning forward or backwards. To help with this, keep your eyes facing forward. Don't look down at the ground right below you; instead, focus your gaze on the ground about 20 feet in front of you.

4. **Check your chin, chest, and shoulders.**

   Keep your chin elevated — not so high that you're looking up into the sky, but lifted so that it's parallel to the ground and not tucked into your neck. Keep your chest lifted and your shoulders back. It should feel rather natural. If you are sticking your chest out too much or raising your shoulders, you may feel a strain in your neck or back. You should feel relaxed, not strained.

### Use your arms as you walk

Now that you're standing with great posture, you want to maintain this position as you walk. To do this, it's important to focus on how you use your arms. If you swing your arms too aggressively, you may find yourself slumping forward and rounding your shoulders, which will put you back in a position of poor posture.

Using your arms correctly, however, can power your walk. In fact, you can even burn more calories — between 5 and 10 percent more — by properly incorporating your arms into your walk.

✔ Start by having your arms hang by your sides with your elbows bent at a 90 degree angle. Hold your hands in a partially closed position, but keep them relaxed. Avoid making a tight fist.

✔ Watch how you move your arms with each step. Your arms should swing back and forth, not diagonally. Your arms should be opposite to your legs. As your left leg steps forward, the right arm should swing forward; then as the left foot steps back, the right arm should go back and the left one should come forward.

✔ As your arms swing forward, watch that they don't swing too high. Your hand should not swing higher than your diaphragm.

You may find using your arms this way tiring at first, and that's okay. Feeling fatigued means your body is working harder and, therefore, burning more calories. Keep at it. You may want to use your arms in this way for just a few minutes at first; then build over time to keep proper arm position throughout the duration of your walk.

# Preventing Walking-Related Injuries

Walking is one of the safest forms of exercise you can participate in. In fact, one of the reasons you've probably selected walking for exercise is its low impact on your body and the decreased risk of injury. So why would you even have to worry about injuries related to walking? The truth is, no matter what you do for exercise, when you move, you have an increased risk for injury. Although your injury risk is much lower with walking than with a high-impact activity like running, you still need to protect yourself and take precautions against injury.

An ache here, a sharp pain there — you may think these little twinges are nothing. But are they really? If you ignore pain, it can turn into a bigger issue. In fact, as many as a quarter million walkers are sidelined each year due to a nagging pain or a walking-induced injury. And although most of these injuries are minor and you can recover and get back to walking again, the damage will have already been done. If you have to take a few days, a week, or even longer off from walking, you lose your routine. Walking is no longer part of your healthy daily habits. You may slip back into old behaviors of becoming more and more sedentary. Your energy levels may start to decline. You may start to see pounds slowly coming back on, and before you know it, you're back to where you started.

This doesn't have to happen to you! By knowing the most common forms of walking injuries, recognizing the signs and symptoms, and knowing what precautions to take to avoid these injuries, you can keep your joints and bones strong and healthy. This way, you won't be sidelined from your walking workout and can continue on your path to achieving your weight-loss and health goals.

# *The most common walking-related injuries*

Any injury to your muscle, bones, or joints can sideline your walking workout for a while. However, certain injuries tend to be more common for walkers than others. Many have even been associated with overuse. Knowing the most common injuries and the signs of each can help you to recognize when you are at risk for developing an injury.

If you notice that you may be feeling a symptom of a common walking injury, don't ignore it! If left untreated, you may end up with a chronic injury that impacts your ability to walk for weeks or even months. Instead, by making a few easy tweaks to your workout, you can continue to walk pain-free.

Following are some common walking-related conditions:

- **Plantar fasciitis:** If you start to feel a tenderness on the bottom of your foot or on your heel, especially in the morning, you could be experiencing plantar fasciitis. The *plantar fascia,* which acts as an arch support and shock absorber of your foot, is a band of tissue that runs from the ball of your foot to your heelbone. When overused through repeated walking and pounding, this band can develop small tears and stiffen, leading to pain. If left untreated, this condition can develop into painful heel spurs as well.

- **Achilles tendinitis:** A pain in the lower calf muscle or the heel can indicate *Achilles tendinitis.* This tendon runs from your heel up to your calf muscle. When overused or irritated, it can become inflamed and cause pain. In severe cases, this condition can be almost debilitating and can even increase the risk of an Achilles tendon tear or rupture.

- **Shin splints:** Tenderness, soreness, or a tightness in your shins can indicate a condition known as *shin splints.* This condition is caused by inflammation in the muscles and surrounding tissues of the lower legs due to constant pounding, such as that of regular brisk walking. Severe pain or a pain in a specific location can also be indicative of a stress fracture in the tibia, so see your physician right away if you suspect this.

- **Bursitis:** If the outside of your hips feel sore, it may indicate a condition known as *bursitis.* The *bursae,* which are fluid-filled sacs that cushion the hip joint, can become inflamed with repeated stress such as the impact from brisk walking. Individuals who have one leg that is slightly longer than the other are more prone to this condition as well.

- **Neuroma:** A pain, numbness, or tingling feeling in the ball of your foot or around your toes can indicate a condition known as *Morton's neuroma.* This condition is caused by a thickening in the tissue surrounding the nerves near your toes. It's typically caused by wearing shoes with too narrow of a toe box, so make sure you wear well-fitted footwear when walking. Also, if you suspect a neuroma, see your podiatrist, as this condition can worsen quickly.

✔ **Runner's knee:** If you experience regular pain or throbbing in your kneecap, you could have what's known as *runner's knee* (which can impact walkers just as much as runners). This condition occurs when the femur bone, which connects your knee to your hip, and kneecap rub together. This rubbing can damage cartilage and increase the risk of tendinitis, both of which can increase pain.

## Reasons for walking-related injuries

Although walking-related injuries are common, they are also quite preventable. When you look at the top walking injuries, many of them have similar causes:

✔ Improper walking technique, such as walking on the inside of the foot

✔ Walking on hard surfaces, such as concrete

✔ Improper footwear, such as footwear with limited padding, footwear that's too narrow or too big, or footwear that provides limited support for arches

✔ Jumping into a walking workout without a proper warm-up

✔ Not building your body up to prepare for your workout (walking at a fast speed before you may be ready, performing a high-intensity walking workout after not walking for months)

✔ Walking on uneven terrain, or uphill or downhill repeatedly

✔ Failure to stretch before and after a walk

✔ Decreased muscle strength in the quadriceps, calves, and hamstrings

As you can see, performing a proper warm-up and cool-down, stretching, and allowing yourself to ease into your walking workout are all key to preventing injuries that can sideline you.

## Preventing injury through proper footwear and equipment

Although little to no equipment is needed to walk for exercise, when you do use equipment, it's vital to use it correctly. Misuse of equipment, the use of poor equipment, or even ill-fitted equipment such as poorly fitted footwear can all increase your odds of developing a walking injury. Some of the most common equipment you may come in contact with when walking for weight loss includes

- ✔ Walking shoes
- ✔ Walking insoles for support
- ✔ Apparel such as socks, sports bras, and visors
- ✔ Ankle or wrist weights for resistance
- ✔ Walking sticks
- ✔ Treadmill

Choosing the right type of equipment and using it in the correct way can actually help prevent injury. For instance, choosing a shoe with a good amount of shock absorption and adequate arch support can help protect against the development of plantar fasciitis. Using a walking stick can help you balance your hips to protect against bursitis and falls. Properly fitted socks can help reduce friction that can lead to blisters. The list goes on and on.

To best protect yourself against injury, make a list of all the equipment you envision yourself using when walking. Now, evaluate each piece of equipment to see whether it can help protect you against injury or whether it may be putting you at a greater risk. Start with your footwear.

Footwear is vital to the protection of your lower body. Poorly fitted footwear can not only increase the risk of foot pain and blisters, but it can also increase the risk of Achilles tendinitis, shin splits, and even neuromas. When choosing footwear, make sure it has the following:

- ✔ **Good arch support:** The type of arch you have can determine the type of footwear you need. If you are flat-footed (low arch), choose a shoe that provides increased stability. If you have high arches, you instead should choose a shoe with neutral cushioning that provides no additional stability. Those with a normal arch can choose just about any shoe; an ideal option would be one providing moderate arch support.

- ✔ **Good shock absorption:** With limited shock absorption, the impact of every step you take travels through your feet and up through your lower body and back. Shoes that provide shock absorption can cut down on the wear and tear your body feels from walking as well as help to prevent against common aches and pains.

- ✔ **An adequate toe box:** One that is too narrow can increase the risk of neuromas as well as blisters. A toe box that's not high enough, and therefore doesn't provide enough room for your toes, can aggravate foot issues such as hammertoes and bunions.

✔ **An adequate width:** The side-to-side fit of your shoe should be snug, not tight. If you have wide feet, ask for a walking shoe that comes in a wide width size. Women with wide feet may want to consider purchasing men's shoes, which are cut larger through the ball of the foot and heel.

✔ **An adequate length:** Make sure there's at least 1/2 inch between your longest toe and the end of the shoe. If not, purchase a larger size.

✔ **Enough life left:** Keep an eye out for signs of wear and tear on your shoes. Older shoes, even if they appear in good condition, may not provide the same support and cushioning.

✔ **The best shoe for you:** Talk to a shoe professional if you're in doubt. Everyone's feet are unique — from the type of arch you have to the size and width of your feet and even your walking needs. If you aren't sure whether a shoe is right for you, ask a shoe professional to help you with your selection for the best possible fit.

For all other walking equipment, evaluate it in the same way. If using a treadmill, make sure it has adequate shock absorption. Also, make sure it has an emergency shut-off switch to protect you from a fall. If you want to use a walking stick, make sure you choose one the appropriate height for your status. When choosing apparel, such as socks, make sure they fit your feet and don't bunch up, which can increase the risk of blisters. The better your equipment is, the safer your walking workout will be.

## Preventing injury through stretching

You know that walking plays a major role in improving health and fitness. However, did you know that stretching can play almost as important a role? Regular stretching is not just important for injury protection, but also for your health. Stretching helps to

✔ Improve flexibility by increasing your range of motion

✔ Improve and correct posture by stretching tight muscles such as hip flexors that pull your body out of alignment.

✔ Increase the flow of oxygen, blood, and nutrients to your muscles and body cells, which can boost energy as well as decrease muscle soreness after a workout

✔ Prepare muscles for a workout and to cool down afterward, protecting against injury

When you walk, you use almost all the major muscles in your body. Brisk walking on unstretched muscles can lead to muscle pulls, tightness, and even injuries such as strains and tears. Stretching on a regular basis, however, helps to improve circulation, and can increase flexibility and decrease

your overall injury risk. When you stretch, you move your joints through a complete range of motion, allowing them to warm up for the workout to come. Some stretches are more beneficial to walkers than others. In this section, I show you the best stretches to incorporate into your walking routine and just when and how to use them.

### Understanding when and where to stretch

Although it may seem like a good idea, stretching cold muscles can actually increase your risk for injury. A brief five-minute warm-up, such as a slow walk, helps to warm up muscles and prepares them for stretching. Once your muscles are warm, you can jump into performing your stretches. Warm muscles are not only less likely to get injured, but they also allow you to stretch further, helping to increase flexibility faster.

A brief stretch of all of your major muscle groups is all that is needed before your walking workout. Stretching out each muscle group, such as your legs, your shoulders, your back, and your neck, allows you to take each muscle through its full range of motion while walking with little risk of a muscle pull or tear. Stretching before your workout can also help to increase circulation, energizing your muscles and allowing you to have more endurance for your walk.

After completing your walking workout, you want to cool down by gently stretching out the muscles you just exercised. The cool-down not only helps your heart rate to return to normal, but can also protect against muscle soreness. When you stop exercising, circulation slows. Without a proper cool-down, blood can pool into body parts, such as the legs, leading to swelling of the extremities. In addition, lactic acid and waste products increase in your muscles during exercise. Stretching helps to mobilize these waste products, cutting down on post-exercise-induced soreness.

### Warming up and stretching

Warming up is essential for any walking workout. A proper warm-up helps to get your blood flowing and prepares your body for the workout that is about to come. Warming up is just what it sounds like: It's a way to increase the temperature in your muscles and joints and increase blood flow to help you stay comfortable while walking and prevent injury.

To start your warm-up routine, begin by walking at a slow, steady pace. You should walk at a pace that feels comfortable to you, but not so slow that you feel no increase in your heart rate. As you walk, you should slowly feel your heart rate elevate and feel a slight increase in respiration.

After this brief five-minute walk, you're ready to begin warm-up stretching before you jump into your full walking workout. As you warm up, you want to incorporate every major muscle group into your stretching routine to enhance flexibility and reduce the risk of injury.

Make sure not to skip the warm-up walk. You never want to stretch a cold muscle, as this can lead to injury.

Your warm-up stretch should start from the top of your body and work its way down, until your entire body is warmed up and ready to jump into your walking workout. Warm-up stretches can all be completed while standing and are dynamic to keep the blood flowing, versus static stretches that you can incorporate into your cool-down to increase flexibility. Here are the basic warm-up stretches to incorporate before you jump into your workout:

- ✔ **Arm circles:** As you walk, hold your arms straight out to your sides. They should be parallel to the floor. Slowly circle your arms in a counterclockwise position (see Figure 6-1). As you circle, begin to increase the size of your arm circles, starting with small circles and ending with larger circles. Repeat this for 30 seconds while walking.

- ✔ **Chest and back extensions:** With arms out to your sides and elbows slightly bent, gently swing your arms across the front of your body (see Figure 6-2). Then swing them back while you open your chest to feel a slight stretch in your shoulders and chest. Your arms should remain parallel to the floor. Repeat for 30 seconds.

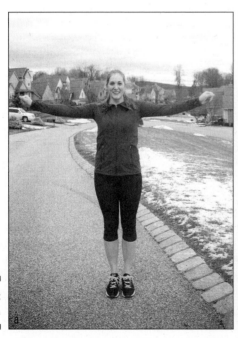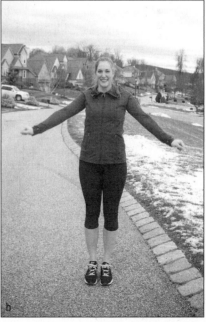

**Figure 6-1:**
Arm circles.

*Photos by Kristen Rath Photography*

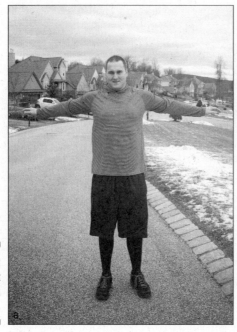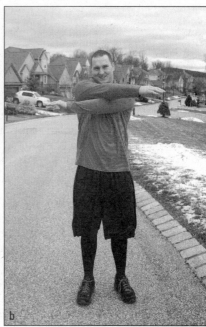

**Figure 6-2:**
Chest
and back
extensions.

✔ **Hip circles:** This exercise should be done while standing, but not while walking. Place your hands on your hips. Keep your core tight and pull your abdominals in. Slowly circle your hips in a clockwise position for 15 seconds (see Figure 6-3). Then switch to circle counterclockwise for 15 seconds.

✔ **Squats:** This exercise helps to warm up all of your leg muscles for the walking workout that's about to come. Stand with your feet shoulder width apart and toes facing forward. Slowly bend your knees to lower your body down, as if you were sitting in an imaginary chair. As you sit, make sure to keep your chest and head up and don't allow your knee to pass over your toe line. Lower your body until your bottom is in line with your knees; then come back up to a stand (see Figure 6-4). Repeat ten times.

✔ **Ankle circles:** This exercise should be done while standing, but not while walking. Stand on one leg and lift your other leg slightly off the floor. Point your toe and gently circle it first in a clockwise direction and then counterclockwise (see Figure 6-5). Repeat this movement with your foot flexed. Now, repeat this stretch on the other leg.

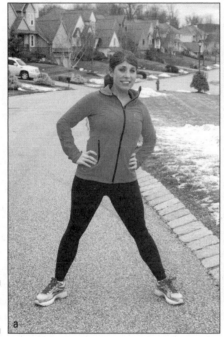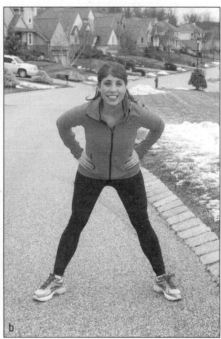

**Figure 6-3:**
Hip circles.

*Photos by Kristen Rath Photography*

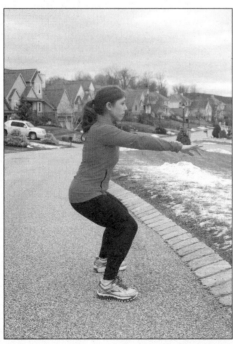

**Figure 6-4:**
Squats.

*Photo by Kristen Rath Photography*

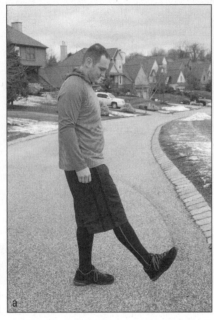
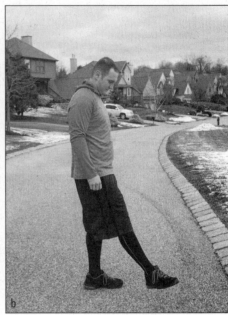

**Figure 6-5:**
Ankle
circles.

*Photos by Kristen Rath Photography*

### Cooling down and stretching

Cooling down after a walking workout is important, as it allows your body to gradually recover from exercise, slow your heart rate, and bring your blood pressure and respiration back to normal. Cooling down gradually versus abruptly stopping a workout may also protect against muscle stiffness after a workout.

To cool down after a walk, you want to slowly reduce the intensity of your workout until you achieve a slow pace at which you feel as though you are breathing normally. Gradually reduce your intensity over a period of a few minutes. If you were walking very briskly, slowly begin to reduce your speed, walking slower each minute, for a period of five minutes. After you have slowed your pace and come to a stop can be a great time to incorporate a post-workout stretch.

Stretching after your workout is ideal, because your muscles are warm and there is less risk of injury. When stretching, remember to start slowly. Don't push your body further than what feels comfortable. If you feel pain, you've stretched too far.

Ease into a stretch until you can feel the muscles being stretched slightly, but you aren't experiencing discomfort. Remember, over time, you can stretch further and increase your flexibility. Too much too soon is a recipe for injury.

When stretching after a walking workout, you want to stretch every major muscle group. Here are the best stretches to incorporate and how to perform each one:

- ✓ **Calf stretch:** Lunge forward while keeping your back heel on the ground. Lean slightly forward until you feel a light stretch in your back calf (see Figure 6-6). Hold this position for 30 seconds; then gently relax your back foot and stand up. Repeat this on the other side to stretch both calves equally.

- ✓ **Hip flexor stretch:** Kneel down with your right knee on the ground and left knee out in front in a lunge position. Your left knee should be bent at a 90-degree angle, making sure that your knee doesn't pass over your toe line. Place your hands on your left knee to help keep your balance. Keep your chest lifted and your chin up. You should feel a stretch in your hip (see Figure 6-7). Hold this position for 30 seconds; then repeat on your other side.

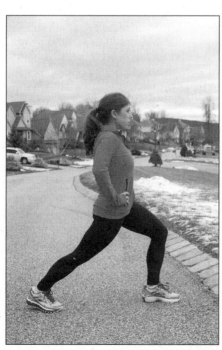

**Figure 6-6:**
Calf stretch.

*Photo by Kristen Rath Photography*

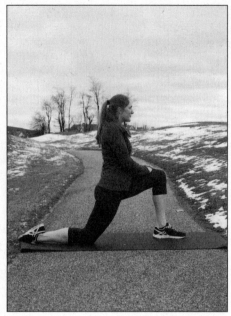

Photo by Kristen Rath Photography

**Figure 6-7:**
Hip flexor
stretch.

✓ **Hamstring and back stretch:** With your feet together and your knees relaxed (not flexed straight), allow yourself to lean forward from your waist. Your arms should extend toward your toes; however, you don't need to reach for your toes. Instead, allow your body to hang under its own weight. Breathe deeply as you lean forward. Allow yourself to reach lower to your toes with each breath (see Figure 6-8). You should feel a stretch in your lower back and your hamstrings. Hold this position for 30 seconds; then slowly roll your back up to a stand.

✓ **Shoulder and arm stretch:** Bring your hands behind your back and interlock your fingers with your elbows bent. Now, slowly straighten your elbows while making sure to keep your chest tall and abdominals in (see Figure 6-9). Straighten your arms as much as you comfortably can (until you feel a slight stretch in your shoulders and biceps). Hold this position for 30 seconds; then slowly bend your elbows and release your hands.

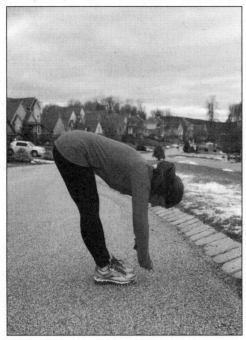

**Figure 6-8:**
Hamstring
and back
stretch.

*Photo by Kristen Rath Photography*

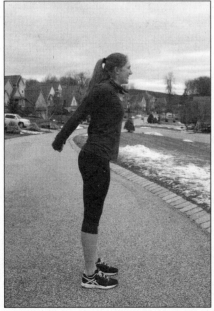

**Figure 6-9:**
Shoulder
and arm
stretch.

*Photo by Kristen Rath Photography*

# Chapter 7

# Fueling Your Walking Workout

* * * * * * * * * * * * * * * * * * * * * * * * * * * * * * * * * * * * * * * * *

## In This Chapter

▶ Seeing how carbs, proteins, fats, and antioxidants affect your walking routine

▶ Fueling your body and keeping your energy high

▶ Targeting belly fat and boosting metabolism

▶ Making sure you get the fluids your body needs

* * * * * * * * * * * * * * * * * * * * * * * * * * * * * * * * * * * * * * * * *

You picked up this book because you want to shed pounds and inches. And you want walking to get you there. It can, and it will! Walking more, even if you make no other change to your diet or lifestyle, will help you to shed pounds. However, if you only walk more and make no changes to your diet, you may see results a bit slower than someone who makes adjustments to his daily food intake. In addition, adding a regular exercise program into your daily routine comes with increased energy and hydration demands.

Knowing how to properly fuel your body before and after your workout will not only help you to lose weight faster, but will help your workouts be even more effective!

## The Impact of Nutrition on Your Walking Workout

When you move, your body requires energy to fuel your muscles and make movement possible. The more you move, the more energy your body needs to keep you in motion. Think of your body in the same way you think of a car. If you want to drive a car, you need to fill its tank with gasoline. The gasoline gives the car the energy it needs to move from Point A to Point B. If you fail to fill the tank, or the tank runs out of gasoline, the car can no longer run. Your body works the same way.

If you don't properly fuel your body and don't refuel it after a hard workout, you won't have the energy you need to continue to move day after day. For this reason, adequate nutrition is vital to your walking workout. If you aren't eating properly, you won't have as much strength, speed, or endurance as you could have, and these deficiencies will impact your overall workout.

The foods you eat (and how much of them you eat) can also significantly impact your weight-loss efforts. Walking more without a change in diet results in a loss of weight. But if you reduce your overall calorie intake while walking, the weight will come off even faster. On the other hand, if exercise increases your appetite and you find yourself eating more, you may see no weight loss at all. That's why focusing on your diet as you increase your overall activity level is helpful in reaching your weight-loss goals.

When it comes to fueling your body for exercise, not all calories are created equal. Calories come from three main *macronutrients*:

- Carbohydrates
- Proteins
- Fats

All are needed by your body; however, each plays a unique role in how it fuels your body. Because each of these macronutrients impacts your body and your muscles in different ways, you want to know just how much of each you need each day, and the best times to consume them, to properly fuel your workout. In addition, food contains micronutrients as well. These smaller nutrients include vitamins, minerals, and antioxidants, which help your body to function in multiple ways. Micronutrients impact everything from muscle contractions to immune system to metabolism and digestion. Making sure you consume the correct amount of both macronutrients and micronutrients each day is vital to good health as well as weight management.

## *Carbohydrates: The good and the bad*

Carbohydrates are the primary source of energy for most types of exercise, including walking. Carbohydrates provide you with the energy you need to achieve peak performance during a workout.

If you want to walk faster, longer, or increase your strength, you need carbohydrates to help you get there. Consuming an adequate source of carbohydrates before and after a workout is vital to keeping your muscles fueled. Eating carbohydrates before a walk gives you the energy to complete the walk. After you finish your workout, eating carbohydrates refuels your body so you have energy stores for your next workout. If you fail to replenish your body's fuel sources after a workout (which are also known as glycogen stores), your body will not have adequate energy reserves for the next workout the following day. In fact, consuming the right type of carbohydrates after exercise not only helps to replenish the fuel you burned, but it can actually help your body to expand the amount of fuel it is capable of storing in your muscles, allowing you to boost your endurance and strength, and therefore maximize your workouts.

Eating too many carbohydrates, however, won't give you even more energy for your walk. Instead, if you consume more carbohydrates than your body needs, your body stores them as excess energy, which means they're stored as fat. Because your main goal is to shed pounds and inches, you want to make sure that you consume the right amount of carbohydrates to maximize your workout, but don't sabotage your weight loss efforts by overdoing it. On average, your carbohydrate intake should make up between 50–60 percent of your total daily calorie intake. The amount of carbohydrates you need to consume before and after a workout will vary depending on the intensity and duration of your walking workout.

A good rule is to consume 15–30 grams of carbohydrate within one to two hours before your workout and then consume an additional 15 grams of carbohydrate for every half hour of exercise within an hour after completing your workout. If your walking workout was a very low intensity workout (a leisurely stroll), you can instead consume 15 grams of carbohydrate for every hour of exercise.

Carbohydrates come from many food sources. They are found in

- Vegetables (both starchy and nonstarchy)
- Fruits
- Milk and yogurt
- Grains and bread products
- Simple sugars

There are two forms of carbohydrates you want to be aware of:

- **Whole-grain carbohydrates:** A whole grain is basically a grain still in its original form, meaning that it contains a bran, an endosperm, and a germ. This makes the grain rich in essential vitamins, minerals, antioxidants, carbohydrates, and fiber. As a result, it is digested slower, preventing blood sugar and insulin levels from spiking. Whole grains also help you feel full longer, making it easier to control your overall daily calorie intake.

✔ **Refined carbohydrates:** Refined carbohydrates are processed, or *refined,* to remove layers of the original grain. Doing this leaves behind all the energy (calories) but little to no fiber, vitamins, minerals, and antioxidants. Some processers add back some vitamins and minerals — that's what's known as an *enriched* grain. However, the enriched grains still don't contain the original amount of antioxidants, fiber, or protein of the whole grain. These grains are typically digested rapidly, spiking blood sugar and insulin levels and causing your body to store fat rather than burn it.

To maximize your walking workout and weight-loss efforts, make sure to choose whole-grain carbohydrates over refined carbohydrates whenever possible.

Because refined carbohydrates elevate insulin levels in your bloodstream, they trigger your body to store more fat — specifically, belly fat. By choosing whole grains that are digested more slowly, you can minimize insulin spikes in your bloodstream and therefore help shed this unwanted fat. In addition, choosing whole grains over refined carbohydrates allows you to experience steadier energy throughout the day. This steadiness helps prevent spikes and crashes in energy that not only impede your walking workout, but can also impact your overall performance throughout the day.

## Supporting your muscles with protein

If you've seen advertisements for body-building supplements, you may think you need to consume insane amounts of protein in order to build any muscle mass or increase strength. However, this really isn't the case. It's true that protein is needed for muscle growth and recovery. When you exercise, especially when you perform resistance exercises such as weight lifting, muscle breaks down. In order for it to rebuild, and become stronger in the process, it needs protein. If you don't take in enough protein through your diet, your muscles will be unable to repair themselves, making increases in strength and muscle difficult.

However, when you exercise moderately, like you will be following the plans in this book, you don't need a large increase in protein. Even athletes' protein needs are only slightly elevated above their nonathletic counterparts. This doesn't mean protein is unimportant, however. To build and maintain muscle (and because muscle helps to make up the majority of your metabolism, you want to maintain it!), you need to make sure you take in an adequate amount of protein to meet your body's daily needs. The average woman needs about 45–50 grams of protein per day while the average man needs about 55–60 grams per day (roughly 15–20 percent of total calories). If you are pregnant or breastfeeding, your needs will be higher (approximately 71 grams per day).

More is not always better when it comes to protein. Protein helps to stabilize blood sugar levels and regulate appetite, so spacing it out throughout the day can be very helpful when trying to lose weight. But consuming much more protein than your body needs doesn't result in muscle being built faster. Instead, excess protein intake just leads to an overall excess of calories being consumed. And excess calories, no matter where they come from, end up being stored as extra fat mass.

## "Fat" is not a four-letter word

Do you panic when you hear the word "fat"? Do you think that eating dietary fat increases your own body fat? If so, think again! Dietary fat is essential for good health. And eating fat doesn't make you fat. Eating too many calories from any macronutrient (carbs, proteins, or fats) makes you gain weight. If you avoid fats all together, you actually may gain weight instead of lose it. Remember the fat-free craze of the '90s? Not many people became skinny from it. Sure, if you reduce your overall fat intake, you may reduce your calories and therefore lose weight. However, many times fat-free foods are filled with carbohydrates and simple sugars, making them less filling. As a result, you get less satisfaction from eating, leading you to eat larger portions and ultimately gain weight.

Fats are critical to your diet for many reasons. They help promote the health of your brain, your skin, your nerves, your hormones, and even your muscles. When it comes to exercise, fats also provide you with the energy you need to complete a long walking workout. If you burn through all of your carbohydrate stores when you exercise, how will you keep going? After your short-term energy is used up, your body turns toward fat stores along with dietary fat to support your increased energy needs during low-intensity exercise, such as walking. Without these dietary fats, you may run out of energy during your workout, leading to you being unable to complete a longer or more intense workout, and therefore burn fewer calories.

Just as with carbohydrates, there are different forms of fats. Choosing the right forms helps you to power through your workout as well as shed pounds:

✔ **Unsaturated fats:** This group contains both monounsaturated fats and polyunsaturated fats. Unsaturated fats tend to be mainly plant-based fats such as oils, nuts, seeds, and avocados. These fats have been found to help decrease inflammation in the body, therefore helping to fight against unwanted weight gain. The majority of the dietary fats you eat should come from this group.

- **Saturated fats:** Saturated fats are mainly found in animal proteins, so a diet rich in high-fat dairy, red meat, and processed meats is high in saturated fat. These fats have been linked with an increased risk for heart disease and elevated cholesterol levels, but most importantly, they may increase inflammation in the body, leading to increased storage of belly fat. A small amount of saturated fat each day is okay, but you want to make sure that less than 10 percent of your total daily calories comes from saturated fat.

- **Trans fats:** Trans fats are found mostly in processed foods such as fried foods, pastries, baked goods, biscuits, muffins, and even some brands of microwave popcorn. These fats can do everything from lowering your good cholesterol to raising your bad cholesterol and triggering inflammation. In fact, research has shown that even just 2 grams of trans fats per day can have a negative impact on your health, so avoiding these is very important. And because these fats can pack inches onto the waistline, you need to eliminate them from your diet to successfully reach your weight-loss goals.

Look out for the words "partially hydrogenated oils" on the ingredient list, as they indicate that a food contains trans fats.

When meal planning, keep in mind that around 25–30 percent of your total calories should come from fat, with 10 percent or less coming from saturated fats (keep your intake of trans fats as close to zero as possible). To fuel your workout as well as shed pounds, aim to fill your diet with mostly unsaturated fats. Within this category, monounsaturated fats and omega-3 fatty acids have been linked with helping to decrease body fat and shrink your waistline. Choosing the majority of your fats from these groups is your best bet. Great sources of these fats include the following:

- **Monounsaturated fats:** Olive oil, canola oil, avocado, olives, peanuts, almonds, pistachios

- **Omega-3 fatty acids:** Fish, shellfish, walnuts, flaxseed, chia seeds

## Amplifying your performance with antioxidants

Vitamins and minerals are essential to overall health, growth, and cell repair and can even impact athletic performance. Some vitamins and minerals play a larger role than others in exercise, but a deficiency or imbalance of any nutrient can ultimately impact your overall performance.

In short, a lack or imbalance of a nutrient can impair optimal health, which over time can begin to impact your body weight as well as your ability to exercise.

One of the reasons that vitamins and minerals have a large impact on overall health is due to their antioxidant properties. *Antioxidants* are essentially chemicals that can slow or prevent damage to a cell. These compounds counteract damaging free radicals (substances that can damage cells) in the body to fight against cell damage. Although there are thousands of antioxidants, some of the most common you may have heard of are vitamins A, C, and E.

So why are antioxidants important for exercise? In addition to being essential to your health regardless of exercise, exercise itself may increase your body's demands for antioxidants. Endurance exercise, such as long-distance walking, can increase oxygen utilization in the body. When this occurs, it can increase the generation of free radicals. Research has shown, however, that regular physical exercise can enhance the body's antioxidant defense system, helping to protect against these additional free radicals created by exercise.

Even though the body has adapted to exercise to protect against free radical damage, you still have to be cautious. The body takes time to make these adaptations. If you are a "weekend warrior" of sorts, exercising intensely once or twice a week but remaining sedentary most days, your body may not adapt as quickly. This is why regular exercise is so important, but in addition, consuming a diet rich in antioxidants is also essential.

The largest sources of antioxidants in your diet are fruits and vegetables. To make sure you consume enough, aim for at least five servings of produce per day. A serving size is equal to:

- ✔ One cup raw or one-half cup cooked vegetables
- ✔ Two cups raw leafy greens
- ✔ One medium piece of fruit (about the size of a baseball)
- ✔ 4 ounces fruit juice
- ✔ ¼ cup dried fruit

Look at your current diet and ask yourself whether you're taking in enough fruits and vegetables. If you aren't, think of easy ways you can add them into meals and snacks. For instance, sprinkle berries on your cereal at breakfast or add a side salad with your sandwich at lunch. Not only will doing this increase your antioxidant intake, but the high-volume, low-calorie nature of fruits and vegetables helps to promote weight loss as well.

# Determining the Right Nutrients to Help You Walk Off the Weight

Knowing which nutrients can help you maximize your workout and weight-loss results is vital. One thing you want to keep in mind while you're walking off the weight is your overall calorie intake. Now mind you, calories alone are not the only thing I want you to focus on. You could eat cupcakes all day long, but as long as you didn't eat too many calories, you'd still lose weight. However, in the process, you'd negatively impact your health, and your strength and endurance during your walks would suffer. That's why you want to make sure you balance your overall intake so you have a calorie deficit to maximize your weight loss while walking, but are still meeting your body's energy and health needs.

Moderation and balance are key when it comes to losing weight through exercise. There's nothing wrong with eating a cupcake occasionally. But the key word is *occasionally.* No food should be off limits completely when you're trying to lose weight. If you're too restrictive, you'll crave more food (and most likely more unhealthy food) than if you allow yourself to splurge occasionally. When you are meal planning, keep in mind my *80/20 rule:* If 80 percent of the time you choose whole, unprocessed foods such as whole produce, whole grains, lean proteins, and plant-based fats, then 20 percent of the time you can fit in a few little splurges here and there.

Use the following rule of thumb when you're placing food on your plate. First, visualize filling at least half of your plate with vegetables and fruits. Doing this ensures you're taking in a good amount of fiber to stay full, along with antioxidants. Then fill one quarter of your plate with lean proteins to build and repair muscle and one quarter with whole grains to boost your healthy carbohydrate intake for energy. Reserving a small place on your plate (one fifth of the plate, or 20 percent) once a day for a little splurge such as a small piece of dark chocolate won't impact your progress too much. Just make sure you keep the splurge small. If portion control isn't your friend, cut back the small splurge to just once a week to prevent it from slowing your results.

## Fueling your body without packing on pounds

In order to lose one pound, you need to burn 3,500 calories. That's a deficit of 500 calories per day to lose one pound per week. Now, if you eat the same amount of calories each and every day and just add walking to your routine, you'll lose weight because you'll be burning more calories. However, not everyone eats the same amount of calories per day. If you burn 300 calories walking one day but indulge in a 500-calorie evening snack, the scale won't be headed in the direction you're hoping for. To help you with this, consider keeping a food journal to track how much you eat each day. Similar to an exercise journal, a food journal can be a great way to know how many calories and nutrients you take in on average, so you can make adjustments if needed to maximize your results.

Although calorie needs vary based on individuals, a physically active woman (following one of the walking plans outlined in this book) can eat between 1,400 and 1,800 calories per day and lose weight. A physically active man can eat between 1,600 and 2,200 calories per day while losing weight. A very active, very tall, or younger individual may be able to eat more and still see a consistent, steady weight-loss rate.

These ranges are just averages and not everyone falls within them. If you want to speed your weight-loss efforts, eating less is not always better. Eating too few calories (typically less than 1,200 calories per day), especially when exercising, results in the slowing of your metabolism, counteracting your weight-loss efforts. In addition, eating too little sets yourself up for extreme hunger and cravings, which can result in binge eating if you aren't careful.

Just as with your walking workouts, ease into dietary changes over time. If you start walking each day, just get adjusted to your new workout first. After a week or two, look at your diet and see whether you may need to make a few adjustments based on your rate of weight loss. If you do, slowly reduce your calories by 100 to 300 calories/day each week until you reach the calorie ranges listed earlier and are steadily losing between 1/2 and 2 pounds per week. When you are balancing out your calories, aim to consume 50–60 percent from carbohydrates, 15–20 percent from protein, and 25–30 percent from fats for a well-balanced diet that promotes health as well as weight loss. This balance allows you to feel satisfied, which fights against hunger and cravings, while reducing your overall calorie intake.

## Promoting weight loss without sacrificing energy

One of the main concerns you may have about altering your current diet while you start an exercise program is a reduction in energy. And those concerns are legitimate. If you don't plan carefully, lowering your overall caloric intake can reduce your energy level, which, of course, results in less energy to walk. And you can see how this pattern can lead to eating less but walking less, thus losing less weight! However, you don't have to suffer from a decrease in energy when adjusting your meal plan. In fact, the exact opposite is possible. Cleaning up your diet can lead to dramatic improvements in energy, which can have you walking longer and faster than you ever thought possible!

As I mention earlier, you can reduce your overall calories and lose weight no matter what you choose to eat. Eat only three 400-calorie cupcakes per day, and the weight will come off. But your energy level (along with your health!) will plummet. Certain foods fuel your body and boost energy much better than others. Within each food group, you find energy boosters along with energy drainers. If you stick to eating mostly energy-boosting foods, you'll find the pounds drop off while your energy soars!

In addition to choosing energy-boosting foods over energy drainers, you also want to make sure to space your calories evenly throughout the day. If you consume a very light breakfast and lunch (or worse, skip a meal) and eat a very large dinner, chances are you'll suffer from reduced energy during the day. Instead, eat a meal or snack including all the macronutrients (carbohydrates, proteins, and fats) every few hours to keep your energy level at its highest.

The following sections show you which foods in various food categories are energy boosters and which ones are energy drainers.

### Vegetables

- ✔ **Energy boosters:** Fresh and frozen vegetables, canned vegetables (low-sodium varieties), 100 percent vegetable juice, vegetables prepared in healthy fats such as vegetables sautéed in olive oil

- ✔ **Energy drainers:** Deep-fried vegetables (for example, French fries, onion straws)

### Fruits

- ✔ **Energy boosters:** Fresh and frozen fruits, fruits canned in juice or light syrup, 100 percent fruit juice, no-sugar-added dried fruit

- ✔ **Energy drainers:** Fruit juice cocktails with added sugar, dried fruit with added sugar, fruit canned in heavy syrup

### Dairy

- ✔ **Energy boosters:** Low-fat milk, yogurt without large amounts of added sugars, cheese (choose lower-fat options or limit full-fat cheese to 2 ounces per day)

> ✔ **Energy drainers:** Large amounts of full-fat milk or cheese, heavy cream, milkshakes, milk drinks with large amounts of sugar, yogurts with large amounts of added sugar (sugar listed in the top three ingredients)

### Grains/Starches

> ✔ **Energy boosters:** 100 percent whole-grain breads, cereals, and pastas; brown rice, quinoa, 100 percent whole-grain pretzels and chips, popcorn

> ✔ **Energy drainers:** Simple sugars such as sugar, syrup, jelly, sugary beverages, and candy; refined carbohydrates such as white bread and white rice

### Proteins

> ✔ **Energy boosters:** Lean proteins including fish, eggs, white meat poultry, lean beef, and lean pork; beans, legumes, nuts, and seeds

> ✔ **Energy drainers:** High-fat animal proteins including bacon, sausage, pepperoni, and salami; large amounts of full-fat cheese

### Fats

> ✔ **Energy boosters:** Plant-based fats such as olive oil, canola oil, avocados, peanuts, almonds, walnuts, pistachios, hummus, oil-based salad dressings

> ✔ **Energy drainers:** Heavy cream, lard, shortening

# Choosing Specific Foods That Promote Weight Loss

What if you could lose an extra inch or two from your waistline just by eating a certain food or drinking a certain beverage? It may just be possible! Just as balance is important as you select the macronutrients that make up your daily diet, the specific foods you choose are also important. Some foods have actually been found in studies to help promote weight loss. The method by which these foods promote a reduction in body fat varies. Some foods may help to rev up your metabolism, while others may maximize your body's ability to burn up fat. Others, just by their powerful anti-inflammatory properties, can reduce stress hormones in the body, therefore fighting against the storage of stubborn belly fat.

So how can you know which foods help to maximize your weight-loss efforts? As I outline for you in the preceding sections, food groups such as lean proteins, fruits and vegetables, and whole grains along with healthy fats can improve health and help in the fight against body fat. However, within each of these food groups, there are certain foods that can have the pounds and inches falling off at a faster rate. The following sections take a look at which foods these are and how to best incorporate them into your daily diet.

# The best foods for burning up belly fat

When you eat certain foods, even with little to no other change in your diet, you can maximize fat loss. For this reason, I call these foods "belly burners." Incorporating these foods into your meal plan a few times per week can help to speed your weight-loss results while you follow your walking plan.

### Blueberries

Blueberries are powerful inflammation fighters thanks to their super-high antioxidant content. But this tasty fruit has another hidden benefit as well: It's a potent belly-shrinker! A study at the University of Michigan Cardiovascular Center found that when rats consumed just 2 percent of their calories from blueberries over a 90-day period, they significantly reduced their percentage of belly fat. Another great benefit was that increasing dietary intake of blueberries was also found to reduce triglyceride levels and increase insulin sensitivity, perhaps cutting risk for cardiovascular disease and diabetes. In addition, they have also been shown to help reduce food cravings, which may help you to stay on track with your weight-loss plan.

### Tart Cherries

Tart cherries are rich in the plant chemical called *anthocyanins*. Not only does this chemical give cherries their bright color, but it also helps burn belly fat.

A study conducted by the University of Michigan found that when mice were given food that contained added cherry powder, their body fat was reduced by 9 percent more than mice fed the same diet without the additional cherry powder. Even better, most of the weight loss came from fat stores in the abdominal area. The mice fed the cherry powder also showed significant decreases in cholesterol levels as well as a decline in inflammatory markers. It's important to note that tart cherries are different from the sweet cherries you may often eat raw. Tart cherries are best found in the frozen food section of your grocery store or dried or in juice form.

### Bell peppers

Bell peppers are an excellent source of vitamin C, which studies have shown helps to return the stress hormone cortisol to normal levels after a stressful situation. When stress levels are elevated, they can mobilize fat stores in your body and reposition them in your midsection. The benefit of eating bell peppers is that after a stressful situation, stress hormones circulate in your body for shorter amounts of time, helping to fight against belly fat storage.

### Whole grains

Foods such as 100 percent whole-grain bread, brown rice, and oatmeal are great sources of whole grains, which have been found to help lower body weight. In addition, research has found that diets rich in whole grains may reduce belly fat and help to reduce overall waist circumference.

### Avocados

Avocados are a great-tasting fruit that is rich in monounsaturated fats as well as potassium. Studies have found that diets rich in monounsaturated fats have been linked with a reduced body weight and reduced waistlines. In addition, diets rich in potassium have been shown to help regulate blood pressure levels, helping to reduce the impact of stress on the body.

### Walnuts

Walnuts are one of the best plant sources of omega-3 fatty acids. These fatty acids are not only strong anti-inflammatory nutrients, but they also help to regulate stress hormones. Elevated stress hormones such as cortisol cause your body to store more fat — specifically, belly fat. However, a diet rich in omega-3 fatty acids can help prevent cortisol levels and other stress hormones from peaking, meaning less of these hormones are circulating in your body, and therefore you start to store less belly fat.

### Cottage cheese

Some research has found that a diet rich in dairy may actually help promote weight loss! A study published in *Obesity Research* showed that obese individuals who ate a diet rich in dairy lost significantly more body fat and weight than other individuals eating the same number of calories but following a low dairy diet. In fact, the dairy-rich diet group lost almost double the amount of fat and weight!

And the best part was a majority of the fat lost came from the midsection. So increasing your intake of dairy may help you to flatten your belly faster than just cutting calories alone.

## The best foods for boosting metabolism

Just as some foods have been found in research to increase your body's ability to shed fat, others have been shown to have a thermogenetic effect on your body. A *thermogenetic* effect is an increase in the amount of energy (calories) your body needs to burn to break down, digest, and metabolize a food. Foods with a thermogenetic effect help to increase your body's metabolism, making you burn more calories throughout the day. The more calories you burn, the quicker you lose weight and the easier it is to keep it off.

The following foods maximize your metabolism:

- **Apples:** This fruit is rich in the flavonoid *quercetin,* which has been shown to block baby fat cells from maturing. It's also a powerful inflammation fighter.

- **Hot peppers:** Rich in capsaicin, these peppers have a thermogenetic effect on the body, boosting metabolism and calorie burn.

- **Ginger:** This spice has been found to have a thermogenetic effect as well as helping to aid in digestion.

- **Green tea:** The main polyphenol, EGCG, in green tea has been shown to have thermogenetic properties as well as help to increase fat oxidation.

- **Red and purple grapes:** These grapes are rich in resveratrol. Studies have shown that resveratrol helps increase metabolism as well as suppress estrogen production, which may help decrease body fat and increase muscle mass.

# Staying Hydrated

When you begin to exercise, you begin to increase the amount of water your body loses through sweat during the day. The intensity of your workout, how long you walk, and the temperature at which you walk all impact the amount of fluid that your body loses.

Staying adequately hydrated is not only essential to your walking workout, but it's also essential to achieving good health and losing weight. Taking in adequate fluids before, during, and after your walking workout can help to boost energy levels as well as metabolism.

To protect yourself against the dangers of dehydration and to maximize your walking workout and weight-loss efforts, make staying hydrated a top priority. How much fluid do you really need? Use the following guidelines when hydrating before and after your walking workout:

- Aim to drink 1 ounce of water per every 10 pounds of body weight within a four-hour timespan before your walking workout. For example, if you weigh 200 pounds, you'll want to consume 20 ounces of water in the four hours leading up to your walk.

✔ Drink 5 to 8 ounces of fluid every 30 minutes during exercise (you may want to increase this amount on very warm days if you're walking outdoors).

✔ To rehydrate after your walk, drink 4 ounces of water for every half hour of walking you completed within two hours after finishing your walk.

The preceding are general guidelines for hydration when exercising. However, hydration needs can vary from person to person and from one workout to the next. To make sure you are adequately hydrated, look at the color of your urine. Clear to pale yellow indicates adequate hydration; however, dark urine indicates dehydration, which means you need to drink more!

By the time you start to feel thirsty, you have already become dehydrated. Slight dehydration can impact your workout by causing your muscles to tire more quickly and decreasing overall endurance. However, in severe cases, when you exercise in hot weather and sweat excessively without properly replacing fluids, dehydration can have a much greater impact. Moderate to severe dehydration can have significant health implications, such as heat exhaustion, dizziness, fainting, and even heatstroke, which can be fatal if left untreated.

# Chapter 8

# Delicious and Healthy Recipes

## In This Chapter

▶ Treating yourself to the best snacks and meals to fuel your body before a workout

▶ Discovering the best snacks and meals to refuel after a workout

n Chapter 7, I outline how critical carbohydrates, proteins, fats, and fluids are to fueling your walking workout. Not only can proper nutrition help to boost energy levels, but it can also help you shed pounds and inches faster, allowing you to see the results you want more quickly. Although you may be aware of the types of nutrients that are best for fueling your body, you may not be sure exactly what foods to choose. And that's where this chapter comes in.

Throughout this chapter, I provide you with recipe ideas that are not only quick and easy, but also maximize your results. Each of the recipes in this chapter contains nutrients that work to maximize your body's ability to burn belly fat, helping to slim your waistline as well as decrease your risk for diseases such as heart disease, diabetes, and even certain cancers.

Each recipe is easy to prepare and tastes great! There's no need to sacrifice taste when losing weight!

# Gearing Up with Good Carbs: Pre-Workout Recipes

To fuel your body for a tough workout, carbohydrates are essential. But not just any carbohydrates — you want to make sure you're fueling your body with whole grains. Refined carbohydrates and simple sugars cause spikes in energy followed by an energy crash. This prevents you from being at your best for the duration of your workout. On the other hand, whole grains are digested more slowly, providing your body with a steady source of energy to maximize your workout potential.

The recipes in this section provide your body with a good source of healthy carbs to help fuel your workout. They're not too heavy in proteins or fats, as these nutrients are slowly digested and may cause you to feel sluggish or cramp up when walking if eaten in large amounts right before your workout. Save these essential nutrients for after your workout instead.

## Fight fat with fat

If you are trying to shed pounds, it may sound like an oxymoron to eat more fat. Eating too much fat will just make you gain more fat, right? Actually, no! Eating the right types of fat can actually help you to shed inches and pounds more easily, all while even improving your health! If it sounds to good to be true, it isn't. Many studies have shown a link between eating a diet rich in monounsaturated fats and omega-3 fatty acids to boost heart health, decrease waist circumference, and even tackle dangerous belly fat.

Planning out your meals and snacks to incorporate good sources of healthy fat every day gives you an advantage when it comes to fighting the battle of the bulge. Monounsaturated fats come mostly from plant-based sources and include avocados, almonds, olives, olive oil, peanuts, pistachios, and hummus. Omega-3 fatty acids are found in plant-based sources such as walnuts, flax seed, and chia seeds and also from fatty fish including salmon and tuna. Aim to incorporate a few servings of healthy fats each day. For instance, try to eat three ounces of fish two to three times per week. Cook with a teaspoon of olive or avocado oil. Snack on an ounce of pistachios or almonds or dip your vegetables into a tablespoon of hummus or peanut butter. By incorporating these healthy fats daily, not only can you reduce your risk of heart disease, but you can also slim your waistline and boost your weight-loss efforts.

# Cinnamon Oatmeal with Almonds

**Prep time:** 2 min • **Cook time:** 35 min • **Yield:** 4 servings

| Ingredients | Directions |
|---|---|
| 3 cups water | *1* Place the water in a saucepan and bring to a boil over high heat. |
| 1 cup steel-cut oats | |
| 2 tablespoons cinnamon | *2* Stir in the oats and allow the mixture to come back to a boil. |
| ¼ cup chopped almonds | |
| 1 teaspoon stevia extract, or zero-calorie artificial sweetener (optional) | *3* When the oatmeal reaches a boil, cover and reduce the heat to medium-low. Let simmer for 20 to 30 minutes, or until the oats reach desired consistency, stirring occasionally. |
| | *4* Sprinkle cinnamon and almonds on top, and add stevia or zero-calorie artificial sweetener, if desired. |

*Per serving:* Calories 140 (From Fat 45); Fat 5g (Saturated 1g); Cholesterol 0mg; Sodium 3mg; Carbohydrate 21g (Dietary Fiber 4g); Protein 5g

*Tip:* When cooking oatmeal, shorter cooking time leads to chewier oats and longer time leads to softer oats.

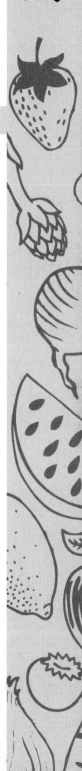

# Rainbow Green Smoothie

**Prep time:** 5 min • **Yield:** 2 servings

| Ingredients | Directions |
|---|---|
| 1½ frozen bananas, peeled | *1* In a blender, combine all the ingredients. |
| 1 frozen kiwi, peeled and sliced | *2* Blend until smooth. |
| 1½ cups chopped rainbow chard, stalk removed | *3* Pour into two chilled glasses and serve each with a straw. |
| ½ cup 100 percent orange juice | |
| 6 ounces nonfat pear or pineapple Greek yogurt | |

*Per serving:* Calories 183 (From Fat 0); Fat 0g (Saturated 0g); Cholesterol 0mg; Sodium 100mg; Carbohydrate 36g (Dietary Fiber 2g); Protein 11g.

# Berry, Rhubarb, and Ginger Smoothie

**Prep time:** 5 min • **Yield:** 2 servings

| Ingredients | Directions |
|---|---|
| ½ teaspoon freshly shredded ginger | **1** In a blender, combine all the ingredients. |
| 1½ cups frozen strawberries | **2** Blend until smooth. |
| ½ cup frozen rhubarb | |
| ⅔ cup 100 percent pomegranate juice | **3** Pour into two chilled glasses and serve each with a straw. |
| ¼ cup nonfat plain Greek yogurt | |
| Dash of cinnamon | |

*Per serving:* Calories 112 (From Fat 4); Fat 0g (Saturated 0g); Cholesterol 0mg; Sodium 23mg; Carbohydrate 25g (Dietary Fiber 3g); Protein 4g.

*Note:* Rhubarb is a tart and tangy fruit that balances out the sweetness of the strawberries.

*Note:* Ginger and cinnamon are two potent belly-blasting ingredients. They add a nice, spicy touch to this smoothie.

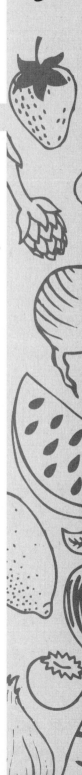

# Frozen Yogurt Bites

**Prep time:** 10 min • **Freeze time:** 25 min • **Yield:** 4 servings

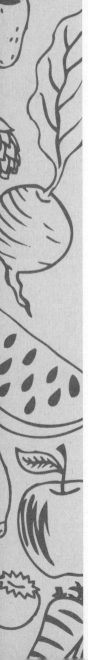

| *Ingredients* | *Directions* |
|---|---|
| **1 cup nonfat vanilla Greek yogurt** | **1** Place the Greek yogurt in a large bowl. |
| **2 bananas, sliced** | **2** Toss the bananas, blueberries, and raspberries into the bowl of yogurt and gently stir to coat. |
| **½ cup blueberries** | |
| **½ cup raspberries** | **3** Line a baking sheet with parchment paper, and place each fruit piece individually on the baking sheet. |
| | **4** Place the baking sheet in the freezer for 25 minutes or until completely frozen. |
| | **5** Peel the frozen fruit from the parchment paper and transfer to a resealable freezer bag; store in freezer until ready to eat. |

*Per serving:* Calories 104 (From Fat 3); Fat 0g (Saturated 0g); Cholesterol 0mg; Sodium 21mg; Carbohydrate 22g (Dietary Fiber 3g); Protein 6g.

*Vary It!* No fruit is off limits! I think mangoes, grapes, pineapples, and peaches would be amazing covered in frozen yogurt!

# Baked Apples

**Prep time:** 3 min • **Cook time:** 10–15 min • **Yield:** 4 servings

| Ingredients | Directions |
|---|---|
| 4 large apples (any variety), cored, peeled, and sliced<br><br>3 tablespoons cinnamon<br><br>1 tablespoon pure maple syrup | *1* Preheat the oven to 350 degrees. Place the sliced apples in an oven-safe glass pan or dish and top with cinnamon and maple syrup. |
| | *2* Bake for 10 to 15 minutes (or microwave for 5 minutes on high power). |
| | *3* The apples should be tender. If they're still firm, bake for 3 to 5 additional minutes in the oven (or 1 to 2 minutes in the microwave). |

*Per serving:* Calories 124 (From Fat 6); Fat 1g (Saturated 0g); Cholesterol 0mg; Sodium 2mg; Carbohydrate 33g (Dietary Fiber 6g); Protein 1g

*Vary It!* Top apples with low-fat whipped cream and, for an added belly-flattening bonus, chopped walnuts.

*Note:* Don't worry about the maple syrup botching your diet. You're only using a small amount, which adds flavor and texture with a minimal blood sugar and insulin response. Aim for pure maple syrup versus brands with high-fructose corn syrup, which may trigger a larger insulin response.

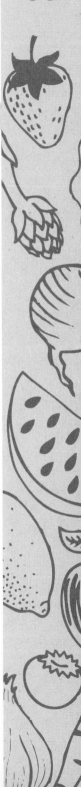

# Crunchy Peanut Butter Banana Bites

**Prep time:** 10 min • **Chill time:** 60 min • **Yield:** 4 servings

| Ingredients | Directions |
|---|---|
| 1 cup 100 percent whole-grain oats | **1** Place the oats in a resealable plastic bag and zip closed. Using a rolling pin, roll over the bag of oats until the oats are small crumbs. |
| 2 medium bananas | |
| 3 tablespoons natural peanut butter | **2** Slice each banana into small, quarter-sized pieces about ½ inch thick. Smear a small coating of peanut butter onto each side of the banana pieces. |
| | **3** Add the peanut butter-coated banana pieces to the plastic bag, and then shake until each piece is coated with the oat crumbs. |
| | **4** Place the coated banana pieces on a plate covered with wax paper. Freeze for 1 hour. |

*Per serving:* Calories 207 (From Fat 65); Fat 7g (Saturated 1g); Cholesterol 0mg; Sodium 46mg; Carbohydrate 31g (Dietary Fiber 5g); Protein 6g.

*Vary It!* If you like, you can skip the freezer and serve immediately at room temperature.

# Belly-Blasting Trail Mix

**Prep time:** 3 min  •  **Yield:** 8 servings

| Ingredients | Directions |
| --- | --- |
| **4 cups high-fiber cereal** | **1** Mix all the ingredients together in a large bowl. Store the trail mix in an airtight container. |
| **¼ cup halved unsalted peanuts** | |
| **¼ cup sliced unsalted almonds** | |
| **½ cup dried cranberries** | |
| **½ cup dried blueberries** | |
| **4 tablespoons dark chocolate chips (at least 70 percent cocoa)** | |

*Per serving:* Calories 190 (From Fat 58); Fat 7g (Saturated 2g); Cholesterol 0mg; Sodium 131mg; Carbohydrate 44g (Dietary Fiber 17g); Protein 5g

*Tip:* This high-fiber, antioxidant-rich mix provides belly-burning monounsaturated fats and is perfect for portioning out into separate containers for an easy on-the-go snack.

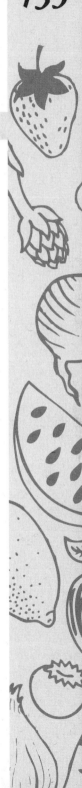

# *Rejuvenating Your Body: Post-Workout Recipes*

After you've worked hard to push yourself through a walking exercise routine, it's time to turn your attention to refueling your body.

The hour after completing your workout is the most essential time to refuel, as this is when your muscles uptake protein the easiest, helping them to repair and grow.

In addition, your body replenishes burned up energy stores within this window so that your muscles will have energy to get them through the next workout.

When you focus on refueling, you want to make sure you're consuming a good source of protein to promote muscle healing and growth. You also want to replenish energy stores so you have the strength and endurance to get through your next workout. But don't get carried away with refueling. If you overdo it, you can take in more energy than you really need, making it challenging to lose weight and keep it off. The recipes in this section help your body refuel and repair, while providing it with nutrients such as omega-3 fatty acids, vitamin C, and whole grains that help you shed belly fat and maximize your results.

# Tropical Yogurt Parfait

**Prep time:** 5 min • **Yield:** 1 serving

| Ingredients | Directions |
|---|---|
| **1 cup fat-free plain or vanilla Greek yogurt** | *1* Place ¼ cup of the yogurt in a clear glass. Top with 1 tablespoon of chopped walnuts and ¼ cup papaya. |
| **¼ cup chopped walnuts** | |
| **1 cup chopped papaya** | *2* Repeat layering the ingredients to make an attractive and tasty parfait. |

*Per serving: Calories 371 (From Fat 178); Fat 20g (Saturated 2g); Cholesterol 0mg; Sodium 90mg; Carbohydrate 27g (Dietary Fiber 5g); Protein 25g*

## Aim for at least 5 a day

If you have heard the phrase "eat 5 a day," you most likely know that it's referring to eating five servings of fruits and vegetables daily. Although you may have known this is important for good health, did you know that eating this amount of produce (or more) daily is essential when it comes to losing weight and keeping it off? Vegetables and fruit are packed full of fiber and nutrients, while low in calories. That's why they are often referred to as "high volume, low calorie foods" — they help to fill you up without filling you out. When you eat more produce, you naturally eat less of other foods, which can make it easier for you to lose weight.

Think about it this way. Let's say you filled your dinner plate with about three cups of pasta, which provides you with about 600 calories. Now, instead, think about filling your plate with three cups of pasta that's been mixed with steamed vegetables. Although your plate visually looks just as full, because you are now eating about one and a half cups of pasta and the rest is coming from steamed vegetables, you have cut the calories of your dish almost in half. Although after eating this dish, you would feel just as full as if you had eaten the pasta-only dish, this dish has much less of an impact on your waistline. In fact, just making this small change every night would result in you losing two and a half pounds in a month! As you can see, adding in your 5 a day can make a significant impact on your weight loss efforts.

Although 5 a day may sound like a large amount, it's pretty simple to fit it in. At breakfast, top your cereal with fresh berries. At lunch, add a cup of vegetable soup and add a side salad to dinner. For a snack, make a fruit smoothie or munch on raw vegetables with peanut butter or hummus. These small changes can lead to big results!

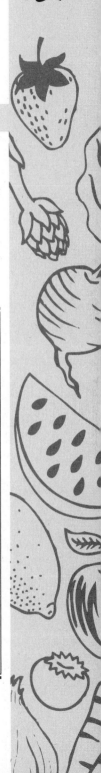

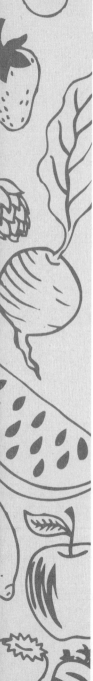

# Veggie-Egg Muffins

**Prep time:** 10 min • **Cook time:** 15–20 min • **Yield:** 8 servings

| Ingredients | Directions |
|---|---|
| **Nonstick cooking spray** | *1* Preheat the oven to 375 degrees and then spray an 8-count muffin tin with nonstick cooking spray. Set aside. |
| **1 tablespoon olive oil** | |
| **¾ cup broccoli, chopped** | |
| **¾ cup diced mushroom** | *2* In a sauté pan, heat the olive oil over medium heat. Cook each of the vegetables separately in the oil until they're tender. |
| **1 cup chopped onion** | |
| **½ cup diced tomato** | |
| **½ cup chopped spinach** | *3* Meanwhile, in a bowl, whisk together the whole eggs and the liquid egg whites. Pour ¼ cup of the egg mixture into each muffin cup. |
| **¾ cup chopped bell pepper** | |
| **4 eggs** | |
| **1 cup liquid egg whites (or 8 egg whites)** | *4* Add one of the following varieties of vegetables and cheese to each muffin cup to make a variety of muffins: |
| **1 cup grated fresh mozzarella cheese** | ½ cup broccoli and ¼ cup mozzarella cheese |
| **¾ cup crumbled part-skim feta cheese** | ¼ cup mushroom, ¼ cup onion, and ¼ cup mozzarella cheese |
| | ¼ cup tomato, ¼ cup onion, and ¼ cup feta cheese |
| | ¼ cup spinach, ¼ cup mushroom, and ¼ cup feta cheese |
| | ¼ cup bell pepper, ¼ cup mushroom, and ¼ cup onion |
| | ¼ cup tomato, ¼ cup spinach, and ¼ cup mozzarella cheese |
| | ¼ cup broccoli, ¼ cup onion, and ¼ cup feta cheese |
| | ½ cup bell pepper and ¼ cup mozzarella cheese |
| | *5* Place the muffin tin in the oven and bake for 15 to 20 minutes. |

*Per serving: Calories 125 (From Fat 68); Fat 8g (Saturated 4g); Cholesterol 106mg; Sodium 281mg; Carbohydrate 2g (Dietary Fiber 0g); Protein 13g*

*Vary It:* The vegetables listed here are just a starting point. You can get creative by substituting different vegetables, different varieties of low-fat cheese, and even lean proteins such as low-sodium ham or turkey bacon.

# Hot and Spicy Vegetarian Chili

**Prep time:** 5 min • **Cook time:** 60 min • **Yield:** 6 servings

| Ingredients | Directions |
|---|---|
| **1 recipe Chili Seasoning (see the following recipe)** | **1** In a large stock pot, add olive oil over medium heat. Add garlic, bell peppers, onion, and celery, and cook until the vegetables are softened, about 8 to 10 minutes. |
| **2 tablespoons olive oil** | |
| **3 garlic cloves, finely chopped** | |
| **1 green bell pepper, chopped** | **2** Add tomatoes, Chili Seasoning (see the following recipe), and 4 cups of water and stir. Allow to simmer over medium heat for 20 minutes. |
| **1 red bell pepper, chopped** | |
| **1 medium green onion, finely chopped** | **3** Stir in the kidney beans, cannellini beans, black beans, and jalapeño (seed the jalapeño if you want less heat to the chili), and allow to simmer for an additional 30 minutes. |
| **3 large celery ribs, chopped** | |
| **One 28-ounce can no-salt-added diced tomatoes** | |
| **4 cups water** | |
| **2 cups red kidney beans, cooked and drained (or one 16-ounce can, rinsed and drained)** | |
| **2 cups cannellini beans, cooked and drained (or one 16-ounce can, rinsed and drained)** | |
| **1 cup black beans, cooked and drained (or one 8-ounce can, rinsed and drained)** | |
| **1 jalapeño, chopped** | |

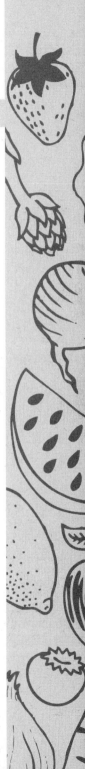

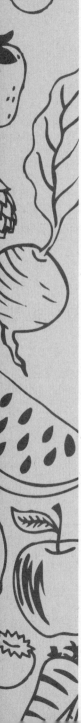

## Chili Seasoning

**1 tablespoon chili powder**

**1 teaspoon turmeric**

**2 teaspoons black pepper**

**1 tablespoon crushed red pepper flakes**

**1 teaspoon garlic powder**

**1 teaspoon onion powder**

**2 teaspoons ground cumin**

**1 teaspoon salt**

**1 teaspoon paprika**

**1 teaspoon dried oregano**

*1* Combine all the ingredients in a small bowl.

*Per serving: Calories 302 (From Fat 55); Fat 6g (Saturated 1g); Cholesterol 0mg; Sodium 488mg; Carbohydrate 50g (Dietary Fiber 15g); Protein 16g.*

# Quick and Easy Turkey Wrap

**Prep time:** 3 min • **Yield:** 1 serving

| Ingredients | Directions |
|---|---|
| **2 tablespoons hummus** | **1** Spread the hummus evenly over the tortilla. |
| **One 12-inch, 100 percent whole-grain tortilla** | **2** Layer the lettuce, tomato, and turkey on the tortilla. |
| **½ cup shredded lettuce** | |
| **½ cup sliced tomato** | **3** Roll the tortilla to create a wrap sandwich. |
| **3 ounces low-sodium, nitrate-free turkey breast cold cut** | |

*Per serving:* Calories 356 (From Fat 59); Fat 7g (Saturated 2g); Cholesterol 71mg; Sodium 251mg; Carbohydrate 42g (Dietary Fiber 5g); Protein 37g

## Meal planning: Lose more weight without hunger

If you think you need to feel hungry to successfully lose weight, think again. Hunger does not help you to lose weight faster. In fact, hunger can actually prevent you from losing weight. Think about the last time you became very hungry. What did you want to eat? It probably wasn't a salad, but instead you probably craved something rich in calories, sugar, or unhealthy fats, like a greasy burger or fried food. When you did get a chance to eat, did you eat nice and slowly? Probably not. Most than likely, if you were ravenous, you wolfed down your food as quickly as you could. That's what allowing yourself to get too hungry does. It leads to less healthy food choices, eating too quickly, and ultimately, taking in more calories than your body needs — promoting weight gain instead of weight loss.

Preventing excess hunger, however, is key to successful weight loss. To do this, it's important to focus on meal planning. Waiting too long in between meals or eating meals with foods that don't fill you will result in hunger. Instead, plan out your meals and snacks so that you aren't going longer than four to five hours with no food. This will allow you to feel ready to eat, but not allow you to get to the point of feeling so hungry you need to gobble up everything on your plate in an instant. To successfully prevent excess hunger and keep weight off, you'll also want to look at what you are eating as well. Foods rich in fiber, lean proteins, and healthy fats take longer to digest, helping you to stay satisfied for longer periods of time. On the other hand, foods rich in refined carbohydrates or simple sugars digest rapidly, leaving you feeling hungry and ready to eat again soon after. For the best success, aim to fill your plate halfway with vegetables and fruit at each meal and then round out the rest of your plate with lean proteins, whole grains, and healthy fats along with low-fat dairy. This balance will keep your hunger at bay while the pounds fall off.

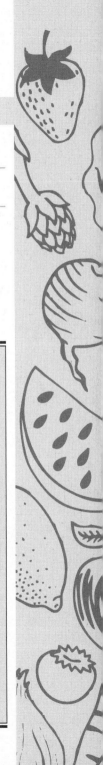

# Whole-Grain Bruschetta Pizza

**Prep time:** 12 min  •  **Cook time:** 15 min  •  **Yield:** 8 servings

| Ingredients | Directions |
|---|---|
| ¾ cup tomato paste | **1** Preheat the oven to 450 degrees. |
| 2 tablespoons minced garlic | |
| 1 tablespoon olive oil | **2** Make the tomato sauce by bringing the tomato paste to a simmer in a small saucepan. Add the minced garlic and olive oil, and allow to simmer for 2 minutes. Remove from the heat and set aside. |
| 16 ounces 100 percent whole-wheat pizza dough | |
| 8 ounces sliced fresh mozzarella cheese | **3** Using a rolling pin, create a 16-inch-diameter pizza from the whole-wheat dough. |
| 1¼ cups fresh bruschetta | |
| 1 cup sliced mushrooms | **4** Spread the tomato sauce evenly over the dough, and then place the fresh mozzarella slices evenly over the sauce. Top the mozzarella with the bruschetta and mushrooms. |
| | **5** Place the pizza on a pizza stone or round pan. Place in the oven and cook for 15 minutes, or until the edges brown slightly. Slice with a pizza cutter into eight even slices. |

*Per serving:* Calories 323 (From Fat 119); Fat 13g (Saturated 5g); Cholesterol 20mg; Sodium 157mg; Carbohydrate 39g (Dietary Fiber 5g); Protein 13g

*Note:* You can purchase the bruschetta and whole-wheat pizza dough at most grocery stores. But, if you prefer, you can make them yourself.

*Vary It!* This recipe only calls for mushrooms, but you can add any toppings you want, such as green pepper, onions, and black olives.

# Smoked Chickpeas

**Prep time:** 2 min • **Cook time:** 20 min • **Yield:** 2 servings

| Ingredients | Directions |
|---|---|
| One 15.5-ounce can low-sodium chickpeas, rinsed and drained | *1* Preheat the oven to 400 degrees. |
| ½ tablespoon smoked paprika | *2* In a medium bowl, combine all the ingredients and coat the chickpeas. |
| ⅛ teaspoon sea salt | *3* Line a rimmed baking sheet with parchment paper and spread out the chickpeas on the baking sheet. |
| ⅛ teaspoon cayenne pepper | *4* Bake for 20 minutes. Allow the chickpeas to cool, and serve. The chickpeas will become crispy as they cool. |

*Per serving:* Calories 171 (From Fat 0); Fat 0g (Saturated 0g); Cholesterol 0mg; Sodium 515mg; Carbohydrate 33g (Dietary Fiber 8g); Protein 10g.

*Vary It!* Like it hot? Turn up the heat by adding more cayenne!

*Vary It!* Replace the spices in this recipe with pumpkin pie spice and vanilla extract for seasonal flavor.

*Note:* Smoked chickpeas are a yummy and nutritious snack filled with protein and fiber to keep you satisfied.

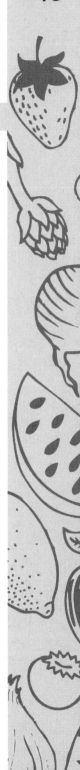

# Sunrise Protein Shake

**Prep time:** 2 min • **Cook time:** 1 min • **Yield:** 2 servings

| Ingredients | Directions |
|---|---|
| 1 frozen banana<br><br>1 cup frozen unsweetened strawberries<br><br>2 tablespoons unsweetened whey protein powder<br><br>1 cup almond milk | *1* Break up the banana into chunks, and place it in a blender along with the strawberries and protein powder. |
| | *2* Add the milk and orange juice to the blender and blend until smooth and creamy. |
| ½ cup 100 percent orange juice | *3* Serve with a straw. |

*Per serving:* Calories 195 (From Fat 29); Fat 3g (Saturated 1g); Cholesterol 30mg; Sodium 129mg; Carbohydrate 34g (Dietary Fiber 5g); Protein 11g.

*Tip:* Whey protein powder is an excellent addition to smoothies. It provides balanced nutrition instead of using only fruit. It also lends a creamier, fluffier texture to smoothies. This protein shake can be enjoyed as an energy-packed breakfast on the go.

*Note:* Frozen fruit is key to smoothie success. When you use frozen fruit, you don't need to add ice, which only waters down the flavor of the drink. Frozen fruit locks in the natural sweetness, too, so you don't need added or artificial sweeteners.

# Part III
# Walking Workouts

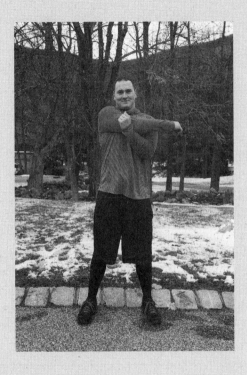

Visit www.dummies.com/extras/walkingtheweightoff for an interesting article.

# In this part . . .

- ✔ Discover what type of walker you are based on your current health and weight-loss goals.

- ✔ Learn the various walking routines available to help increase weight loss, shed inches, and improve overall health.

- ✔ Maximize your walking workout with new techniques and equipment for the fastest results.

- ✔ Delve into the causes of weight-loss plateaus and figure out how to break through them to achieve your ultimate weight-loss goals.

# Chapter 9

# Creating the Best Walking Routine for You

## In This Chapter

▶ Setting your walking workout goals

▶ Figuring out what type of walker you are

▶ Choosing a walking plan that fits your goals

▶ Assessing your walking level and getting started

*W*alking can offer many wonderful benefits. From losing weight to toning muscles and even boosting metabolism, walking has something to offer everyone. And now it's time to get started! In order to be as successful as possible with your walking plan, you want to determine a few things about yourself:

✔ What are your goals for wanting to walk?

✔ What type of walker are you?

✔ What is your walking level?

This chapter helps you answer all of these questions and shows you how your answers can help you mold a successful walking plan. Whether you're just getting started or are a seasoned exerciser, you can select a walking plan that meets your needs and gets you to achieve your goals quickly and easily.

## Setting Your Walking Workout Goals

If you picked up this book, you're no doubt interested in starting a walking workout for weight loss. However, the reasons for wanting to lose weight or choosing walking as a means to achieve that goal may vary from person to person. Perhaps you were just diagnosed with diabetes and want to lose weight to control your health. Or maybe you used to be an athlete and have become sedentary and want to get moving again. Or maybe you've never exercised and want to start, and walking seems like the best choice for you. Whatever your reasons, a walking workout can offer benefits to everyone. You just need to understand how walking can get you to where you want to be.

Personal goals for walking tend to fall into a few main categories:

- ✔ **Walking to achieve weight-loss goals:** In this category, you may set a goal for yourself to lose a set number of pounds, such as losing 20 pounds. Or you may set a goal to lose inches, such as reducing your waistline by 3 inches.

- ✔ **Walking to achieve health goals:** Here, you may set goals for yourself to improve health, such as to lower cholesterol, blood pressure, or blood sugar levels. You may also set preventative health goals here, such as walking to reduce your risk of cancer or heart disease.

- ✔ **Walking to achieve fitness goals:** If you're interested in feeling stronger, having more endurance, and boosting energy, your walking goals are related to fitness. Here, you may set a goal such as being able to walk a mile in under 15 minutes or being able to walk uphill for a certain amount of time or distance. You may also set a fitness goal to cover a certain distance, such as completing a 5k (5-kilometer walking event).

- ✔ **Walking to achieve mental health/stress reduction goals:** If you have a high stress level, you may walk to help calm your nerves, improve your sleep habits, or even just to enjoy time with your spouse or a friend or family member. Taking even a few minutes away from the stresses of work or family life to clear your mind can be a goal that not only rejuvenates you, but improves your long-term health as well.

When you are looking at your reasons for wanting to walk for weight loss, you may have just one goal, or you may have goals for yourself in each of these categories.

It's a great idea to have multiple goals. For instance, if one week you find your weight loss progress slowed, but at the same time you notice a drop in your pants size or find that your blood pressure has decreased, these accomplishments can keep you motivated as you work toward achieving your other goals.

# How your walking goals impact your workout

After you've determined your reasons for walking and your goals, take out a piece of paper and write down each goal. Now, look at that list and ask yourself, "Which of these goals is my main focus?"

Prioritize your goal list so you know which goals are most important to you. Once you can see which goals mean the most to you, you can use these goals to help shape and mold your walking routine:

✔ **If weight loss is your top goal:** Focus on creating a walking routine in which you not only walk for a set distance or duration each day, but also work on increasing your overall daily steps.

✔ **If toning and losing inches is your top goal:** Make sure your walking routine incorporates resistance training to strengthen and tone muscles as well as interval training to help shed belly fat and inches.

✔ **If improving health is your top goal:** Focus on increasing your overall daily movement and decreasing the amount of time you are sedentary each day.

✔ **If decreasing stress is your top goal:** Make sure you choose a relaxing walking location and create a plan that you look forward to every day.

✔ **If boosting your fitness is your top goal:** Make sure your walking routine challenges you each day by making you strive to increase your speed, your walking distance, your strength, or a combination of these.

# How your health impacts your walking goals

When setting goals for yourself, you want those goals to push you, but you also want to make sure they are realistic and achievable. The worst thing you can do to yourself is to set goals that are too high or unattainable. This tactic only sets you up for failure and disappointment, which may discourage you from exercising at all.

Wanting to challenge yourself and think big when it comes to goal setting is perfectly understandable. However, remember that you can always readjust your goals and set additional goals for yourself. Focusing too much on large, long-term goals or goals that may be unrealistic is more discouraging than encouraging. You also need to think about your current health and how it impacts what you are able to do and achieve when it comes to exercising. Certain health conditions may limit your walking plan. This doesn't mean that you can't walk or lose weight and boost your fitness level. However, it may mean that you have to make a few adjustments to your plan to make sure it's appropriate and safe for you.

No matter your age, your current health condition, or your fitness level, walking to lose weight can work for you. However, making sure your goals match your needs and customizing your walking plan for your individual requirements helps you to be more successful in the long run and achieve your long-term goals more quickly!

### Start slowly

No matter what your age, if you've never exercised before or haven't exercised anytime in the last six months, you need to start slowly. You should first consult your physician to be cleared for exercise. After you've been cleared, you need to realize that it takes time to build strength and endurance. Start out by setting smaller distance or time goals for yourself and increase your goals as these become achievable. You may want to focus on walking for short bursts a few times per day instead of all at once and building up to a long walk as your endurance increases. Starting out walking too much too quickly can increase your risk for burnout and injury.

### Be mindful of your existing health conditions

If you have a health condition such as heart disease or diabetes, you need to take extra care when designing and implementing your walking routine. Chapters 12 through 16 outline how to adjust your walking routine based on these conditions as well as pregnancy, osteoporosis, and osteoarthritis. With all of these conditions, walking can be very beneficial to your health, but you still must take certain precautions. For instance, if you have osteoporosis, you need to decrease your risk for falls by avoiding uneven terrain to guard against fractures.

If you have diabetes, you need to take extra care to protect your feet and check them after each walk to avoid wounds that are difficult to heal.

## What Type of Walker Are You?

When it comes to walking, there are many different types of "walking personalities." Understanding your walking personality can help you select the best walking plan for yourself long term.

If you select a walking plan that matches your personality, you are less likely to become bored or lose motivation. You're more likely to stick with your plan day in and day out, achieving your goals more quickly as well as maintaining your results long term. Take a look at some of the most common walking personality types:

- ✔ **"Getting down to business" walker:** Your time is precious and you don't want to waste any of it. You want an efficient walking workout that maximizes every minute to achieve the most results in the shortest amount of time.

- ✔ **"Taking it all in" walker:** You have a relaxed personality when it comes to working out. You prefer to walk for enjoyment at your own pace and take in your surroundings.

- ✔ **"Hesitant" walker (walking because you have to):** You realize you need to exercise for your health and to lose weight, but may feel resistant to doing so. You have selected walking because it seems like the easiest and most practical form of exercise. You've made the commitment to walk but are doubtful that you'll enjoy it.

- ✔ **"I love to walk" walker:** You walk for the love of it rather than for exercise. You love to walk, to see the sights, and to stay active. For you, the weight loss and health benefits of walking are just an added bonus.

- ✔ **"Squeeze it in when I can" walker:** You have a busy schedule and don't have much time for a structured exercise routine. You have determined, however, that you can increase your overall daily steps and fit in small, short walks throughout the day to help you burn calories and improve your health.

Do you recognize yourself in one of these walking personalities? The type of walker you are influences the walking plan you select for yourself. For instance, a "getting down to business" walker wants a high-intensity plan that he can schedule into his day for a set amount of time, whereas a "hesitant" walker would be scared away by such a plan. Instead, this type of personality would do better with a walking plan that focuses on taking small, short walks throughout the day, as would the "squeeze it in when I can" walker.

Recognizing what you want from your walking plan along with your walking personality is vital in your selection of your workout routine. Knowing that your goals and personality match your plan helps you to not only be successful but to also reach your goals quickly and easily.

# Using Your Goals to Select Your Plan

Your goals determine how you walk, when you walk, and even the intensity of your walk. Matching up the correct walking plan with your needs guarantees you'll be successful with your weight loss and health goals. The following sections take a look at the type of walking plans you may select from and which personalities are the best fit for each plan.

## Power walking to increase stamina

If your main goals are to increase endurance, build speed and strength, and improve your overall fitness level, then you want to make sure your walking plan allows you to achieve these goals. A walking plan that allows you to increase the duration of your walks and speed over time is essential. In addition, a walking plan that varies your terrain by adjusting your incline level can help to further improve stamina and strength. Interval training can be an essential component of such a workout to help you achieve your fitness goals.

## Leisurely walking to decrease stress

Walking to reduce stress is just about getting up and getting moving. Both high-intensity, brisk walking and a leisurely stroll can reduce stress levels and clear your mind. If you want to conquer stress while shedding pounds and inches, adding some power walking to your fitness routine will allow you to reach your goals faster. However, just the act of reducing stress can help to lower body weight and belly fat. So even if you choose a less intensive workout routine, such as taking a relaxing stroll around the block at lunchtime each day, this type of walking will still help to lower fat-storing stress hormones. In addition, anytime you get up and get moving, you are working to burn additional calories and drop weight.

## Walking to maximize health

Walking helps to improve circulation, decrease stress levels, lower blood pressure and blood sugar, and reduce the risk of many diseases. Research has shown that even small amounts of walking, just a few minutes a day or a few miles per week, can have a dramatic impact on overall health and disease prevention. No matter how you walk or how often, whenever you walk you are improving your health. However, depending on your health needs, you may want to adjust your walking plan to gain the best benefits. If you've been diagnosed with insulin resistance (a precursor to type 2 diabetes), weight loss and a reduction in belly fat are essential in helping to prevent diabetes. In this situation, adding resistance or interval training to your walking workout can maximize your fat loss and help you to more quickly achieve your long-term health goals.

## Walking to shed pounds

If your main goal above all else is to lose weight, then you want to focus on a walking plan that incorporates two things: increasing your overall daily movement and adding a structured walk that incorporates resistance and/or interval training. This combination ensures that you are burning more calories all day long, increasing your overall movement each day, and working to boost your body's metabolism and fat-burning ability.

## Walking to burn up belly fat

Maybe you are at a healthy body weight, but your waistline is still wider than you'd like. Or perhaps you tend to hold excess weight mainly in your belly. As much as you may want to banish belly fat for appearance reasons, reducing belly fat is vital to your health. Excess levels of belly fat can increase your risk of everything from heart disease to diabetes and even certain cancers. Interval training has been found to be one of the most effective strategies for burning up this stubborn fat. Incorporating a walking routine with an emphasis on interval training is key to your success.

# Determining Your Walking Level and Getting Started

The biggest concern with trying to start an exercise program that's too challenging is that it can be discouraging. If your exercise plan is more discouraging than encouraging, it can be hard to talk yourself into doing it. If it's a struggle to make yourself walk each day, you're not likely to stick to your routine long term. And no matter how great an exercise program is, if you aren't consistent with it, you won't see results.

Conversely, if you've already been exercising for a while, you need to assess your current fitness level compared to the walking plan you'd like to start. Make sure the plan you choose for yourself at least matches the intensity of your current exercise routine and will provide you with some challenge. If your walking routine is too easy for you, you may not burn as many calories or as much fat as you hope to, which will slow your results. In addition, an exercise routine that doesn't challenge you may become boring over time, making it hard to stick with.

If you've been running 3 miles per day but your knees can no longer take the pounding, switching to a walking routine is a great option. However, if you switch to walking only 1 mile per day, you may notice a decline in your endurance level as well as the amount of calories you burn each day. To prevent this, you can aim to walk the same distance, or you can increase the intensity of your walk by adding an incline or resistance. This way, your workout still provides your body with a challenge and continues to enhance your fitness level while working to help you shed pounds and inches (but without all the pounding on your joints!).

## Getting started as a beginning walker

You may want to classify yourself as a beginning walker if you

✔ Have not participated in structured exercise before

✔ Have not been physically active on a regular basis for the past six months or longer

✔ Feel easily winded or fatigued after walking for a few minutes

✔ Struggle with walking long distances or uphill/up stairs

✔ Feel nervous about starting an exercise routine

✔ Are coming back from an injury that left you unable to be physically active for a period of time

✔ Have a health condition that restricts you from exerting yourself physically or have restrictions on elevating your heart rate

If you are new to exercise or to walking, it's normal to feel some reservations about getting started. You may be nervous about fitting regular exercise into your daily routine. Or perhaps you are concerned about challenging your body too much too soon. It's very common to feel this way, and you aren't alone. In fact, almost everyone who has started an exercise routine experienced all the same feelings and concerns at some point. When it comes to exercise, there's really no secret as to what you need to do. If you listen to your body and ease into walking slowly, you can work toward achieving all your goals.

In Chapter 10, you see all the various walking routines you can participate in to help you achieve your weight loss and health goals. Depending on your fitness level, some plans will be more suited for you than others. If you've never exercised before or are very hesitant about getting started, consider starting with the walking routine to increase daily activity at first. This plan helps you to increase your overall level of movement during the day. Once you gain confidence with your ability to be more active, you may choose to challenge yourself and your body by moving on to a plan to maximize your weight loss or fitness level.

## *Getting started as a seasoned walker/exerciser*

You can identify yourself as a seasoned walker or seasoned exerciser if

- ✔ You are already consistently walking or exercising for at least 20 minutes a day, two times per week or more
- ✔ You can walk for long distances without becoming tired or winded
- ✔ You are confident in your ability to exercise
- ✔ You have found ways to work exercise into your daily routine and stick with it
- ✔ You enjoy exercise and look forward to completing a workout and the benefits it provides
- ✔ You have been exercising on a regular basis, but feel your results have plateaued

If you have walked for fitness in the past or are already walking for fitness, you'll want to examine your goals and how your fitness routine is helping you achieve them. If currently you walk for 20 minutes daily at a casual pace but haven't seen the scale moving in the right direction, it's time to change your workout. With walking, it's easy to adjust your workout to maximize your results. In Chapter 10, you see just how easy it is to do this by reviewing the various walking plans.

Anything extra you can do each day will help you to achieve your goals faster. If you increase the duration of your walk, how quickly you walk, how much resistance there is on your walk, and so on, you'll start to see results faster. By making tiny tweaks to your current walking routine, you can dramatically improve your weight-loss efforts and health.

Even if you are following a structured walking routine on a regular basis, you'll still want to pay close attention to your overall daily physical activity level. As I mention earlier in this book, research has found that individuals who go to the gym and work out for an hour a day but are mostly sedentary the remainder of the day expend less energy (which means they burn fewer calories) during the day than those who don't exercise but are mostly active the majority of the day. That's why making sure you are up and moving more, in addition to scheduling walks, is vital to your success.

# Chapter 10

# Walking Routines

· · · · · · · · · · · · · · · · · · · · · · · · · · · · · · · · · · · · · · · · · ·

· · · · · · · · · · · · · · · · · · · · · · · · · · · · · · · · · · · · · · · · · ·

*B*efore delving into this chapter, you'll want to figure out what type of walker you are, what your main goals are for your walking workout, and whether you prefer to walk indoors, outdoors, or a combination of both. (If you haven't done so already, check out Chapter 9 for more info on walking types and goals, and Chapter 4 for the ins and outs on walking indoors versus outdoors.) Once that's out of the way, it's time to put your feet where your mouth is and start getting down to business!

This chapter outlines a variety of walking programs. You can stick with just one program until you reach your goals, or you may opt to switch between programs as your goals and results change over a period of time.

As you read this chapter, you'll notice that I characterize walking in two ways: as walking plans and walking programs. Here's the difference:

- ✔ **Walking programs:** Walking programs provide a complete outline for your walking workout from week to week, based on your goals. For example, the weight-loss maximizer program helps you shed pounds and inches the fastest, while the stress reducer program focuses more on lowering your overall stress level and improving your health. Remember, at any time, you can switch your walking program if you feel you decide to change your goals or the focus of your workout.

- ✔ **Walking plans:** Walking plans make up the walking programs. To help you gain the fastest results and make your walking program as effective as possible, you don't want to repeat the same walk day after day with no variation. That's why I've created walking plans that are meant to be mixed into your walking program throughout the week. These plans focus on everything from toning muscles to increasing endurance and even lowering stress. Depending on the walking program you choose, you'll incorporate some of these plans more often than others.

# Deciding on a Walking Program

Since you've picked up this book, no doubt you want to lose pounds and inches. However, how you lose weight and the additional goals you have for yourself as you lose weight can help to determine just which walking plan is best for you:

- **Weight-loss maximizer program:** If you want to shed the maximum number of pounds and inches, this program is for you. A combination of interval training, resistance exercises, and brisk walking helps you to banish stubborn belly fat and torch calories.

- **Fitness enhancer program:** As you lose weight, you may want to increase your overall strength or improve your endurance and speed. This program can get you there! This total body workout challenges and strengthens your muscles to improve both your speed and your stamina.

- **Stress buster program:** Elevated stress levels can pack on the pounds and expand your waistline. By increasing your overall daily movement and working to reduce stress levels, you can not only lower your overall body weight, but you can reduce the most dangerous fat — belly fat!

- **Disease fighter program:** If the main reason you have decided to lose weight is to help prevent or control disease, then this is the program for you. Not only does this program help you lose weight, but it also helps to improve your overall health, strengthen your cardiovascular system, and decrease your risk for diseases such as diabetes and even certain cancers!

- **Managing menopause program:** If you have noticed the scale creeping upwards or your waistline expanding with the start of menopause, you don't have to just accept these changes. This walking routine will help to turbocharge your metabolism (which becomes more sluggish with menopause) helping you to get your old body back in no time!

- **Boosting daily activity program:** If you move more and eat the same (or less), you'll lose weight. If right now you are mostly focused on just moving more throughout the day without scheduling a set time for exercise, this program is perfect for you. By tracking your overall daily movement, this program helps you burn additional calories and shed pounds, and keeps them off long term.

Always make sure to consult your physician before starting or changing any exercise routine.

# The Walking Plans That Make Up the Programs

The walking plans in this section are the framework for building each of the walking programs I outline in more detail later in this chapter. These walking plans challenge your body, torch calories and fat, tone your muscles, and boost metabolism. The way these walking plans are combined and incorporated into the walking program you choose is what helps you see results quickly and easily.

Each walking plan incorporates a brief warm-up and cool-down period. Stretching at the end of each workout is also recommended. See Chapter 6 for detailed descriptions and images of the best stretches to incorporate into your walking workout.

Each of the walking plans contains three levels. Level 1 is the easiest level and Level 3 is the most challenging. As you look at your walking program, you'll see that most programs incorporate Level 1 and Level 2 in the earlier weeks of your walking program. By the end of your walking program, you'll be incorporating mostly Level 3 plans.

Before you look through the various walking plans, however, you need to become familiar with the terminology for the types of walking that the plans incorporate. First, I bring you up to speed regarding the types of walking you need to know about; then I describe each of the plans in detail.

## Types of walking

There's more than one way to walk. You need to spend a little time warming up at the beginning of each walk and cooling down at the end. In between, you can walk at a variety of speeds, or paces, which vary the intensity of your workout. The following sections describe each of these types of walking.

### Warm-up walking

The objective of warm-up walking is to get your blood flowing and your muscles prepared for a more intensive workout. Your pace during a warm-up walk should be slow and steady. The intensity level is one at which you should be able to carry on a conversation if you want to.

### Cool-down walking

Similar to warm-up walking, cool-down walking after a workout allows you to slow your heart rate back to normal. It also gives your muscles time to wind down. If you just sit down after completing a workout, your muscles are more likely to stiffen and cause soreness. During the cool-down walk, you should gradually slow your pace from a moderate walk to a slow, casual walk.

### Moderate walking

Think of a speed between window shopping and power walking, and you'll find moderate-pace walking. At this speed, you should comfortably be able to speak a sentence or two, but become winded carrying on a full conversation. You should walk at a faster pace than your normal day-to-day walking speed, but not so fast that you feel out of breath.

### Brisk walking

One step up from moderate-pace walking is brisk walking. At this speed, you should be able to say a few words or a brief sentence, but talking in full sentences should leave you winded. You should feel that you are pushing yourself to walk at a slightly faster pace than normal; however, this should still be a speed you can walk at for a good amount of time.

### Fast walking

Now you're at power-walking speed. This is a face-paced walk where you can say a word or two, but can't speak a full sentence. This is also a speed that you have to push yourself to achieve. You should be able to walk at this pace for a period of minutes, but not for a long duration.

### Very fast walking

Walking at a very fast pace is walking as fast as you can possibly go. You should only be able to maintain this speed for a minute or less, but you really want to push yourself here. Use your arms and your core, and propel yourself as if you were race walking!

### Casual walking with deep breathing

When you walk for enjoyment or walk with a friend and chat, you're walking at a casual speed. You're walking to increase your movement, but not to challenge your endurance. Your heart rate and breathing may increase slightly, but you should be able to carry on a conversation. During this walk, you want to include what's known as *belly breathing*. To do this, first practice this breathing activity when you are still and not walking. Once you're comfortable with this, incorporate a few deep belly breaths every few minutes during your walk to help fight stress. See Figure 10-1 for an example of belly breathing.

To practice belly breathing, follow these steps:

1. **Start by sitting or lying in a comfortable position.**

2. **Place one hand on your chest and the other just below your ribs on your belly.**

3. **Take in a deep breath through your nose.**

   Breathe in deeply enough that the breath forces your belly to push your hand out. Your chest should not be moving as you do this.

4. **Now exhale through pursed lips (as if you're trying to whistle).**

   As you breathe out, focus on feeling the hand on your belly go in.

5. **Repeat Steps 3 and 4 five to ten times, breathing in slowly and deeply.**

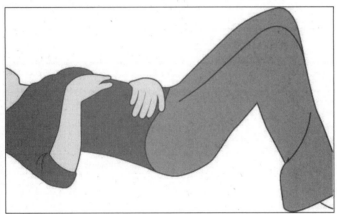

**Figure 10-1:**
Belly
breathing.

## Interval walking plan

Th interval walking plan incorporates interval training to help boost the calorie and fat burn of your walking workout. This plan is outlined in Tables 10-1 to 10-3.

| Table 10-1 | Interval Walking Plan, Level 1 |
|---|---|
| *Time* | *Walking Type* |
| 0–5 min. | Warm-up walking |
| 5–10 min. | Moderate walking |
| 10–11 min. | Fast walking |
| 11–15 min. | Moderate walking |
| 15–16 min. | Fast walking |
| 16–20 min. | Moderate walking |
| 20–21 min. | Fast walking |
| 21–25 min. | Moderate walking |
| 25–26 min. | Fast walking |
| 26–30 min. | Moderate walking |
| 30–35 min. | Cool-down walking |

| Table 10-2 | Interval Walking Plan, Level 2 |
|---|---|
| *Time* | *Walking Type* |
| 0–5 min. | Warm-up walking |
| 5–7 min. | Moderate walking |
| 7–8 min. | Fast walking |
| 8–10 min. | Moderate walking |
| 10–11 min. | Fast walking |
| 11–13 min. | Moderate walking |
| 13–14 min. | Fast walking |
| 14–16 min. | Moderate walking |
| 16–17 min. | Fast walking |
| 17–19 min. | Moderate walking |
| 19–20 min. | Fast walking |
| 20–22 min. | Moderate walking |
| 22–23 min. | Fast walking |
| 23–25 min. | Moderate walking |
| 25–26 min. | Fast walking |
| 26–28 min. | Moderate walking |

| Time | Walking Type |
|------|--------------|
| 28–29 min. | Fast walking |
| 29–31 min. | Moderate walking |
| 31–32 min. | Fast walking |
| 32–34 min. | Moderate walking |
| 34–39 min. | Cool-down walking |

| Table 10-3 | Interval Walking Plan, Level 3 |
|------------|-------------------------------|
| **Time** | **Walking Type** |
| 0–5 min. | Warm-up walking |
| 5–6:30 min. | Moderate walking |
| 6:30–7:30 min. | Fast walking |
| 7:30–8 min. | Very fast walking |
| 8–9:30 min. | Moderate walking |
| 9:30–10:30 min. | Fast walking |
| 10:30–11 min. | Very fast walking |
| 11–12:30 min. | Moderate walking |
| 12:30–13:30 min. | Fast walking |
| 13:30–14 min. | Very fast walking |
| 14–15:30 min. | Moderate walking |
| 15:30–16:30 min. | Fast walking |
| 16:30–17 min. | Very fast walking |
| 17–18:30 min. | Moderate walking |
| 18:30–19:30 min. | Fast walking |
| 19:30–20 min. | Very fast walking |
| 20–21:30 min. | Moderate walking |
| 21:30–22:30 min. | Fast walking |
| 22:30–23 min. | Very fast walking |
| 23–24:30 min. | Moderate walking |
| 24:30–25:30 min. | Fast walking |
| 25:30–26 min. | Very fast walking |
| 26–27:30 min. | Moderate walking |
| 27:30–28:30 min. | Fast walking |

*(continued)*

**Table 10-3** *(continued)*

| Time | Walking Type |
|------|--------------|
| 28:30–29 min. | Very fast walking |
| 29–30:30 min. | Moderate walking |
| 30:30–31:30 min. | Fast walking |
| 31:30–32 min. | Very fast walking |
| 32–37 min. | Cool-down walking |

## Speed walking plan

The speed walking plan, outlined in Tables 10-4 to 10-6, maximizes the speed at which you walk. By walking more quickly, you can burn more fat and more calories with each minute of your walking workout.

When you start with Level 1, record the number of steps you take. When you move on to Level 2, increase your speed so that you can cover 500 more steps in the same time. At Level 3, increase your speed so that you're covering 1,000 more steps than you were at Level 1.

| Table 10-4 | Speed Walking Plan, Level 1 |
|------------|------------------------------|
| Time | Walking Type |
| 0–5 min. | Warm-up walking |
| 5–40 min. | Brisk walking |
| 40–45 min. | Cool-down walking |

| Table 10-5 | Speed Walking Plan, Level 2 |
|------------|------------------------------|
| Time | Walking Type |
| 0–5 min. | Warm-up walking |
| 5–40 min. | Brisk walking |
| 40–45 min. | Cool-down walking |

| Table 10-6 | Speed Walking Plan, Level 3 |
| --- | --- |
| *Time* | *Walking Type* |
| 0–5 min. | Warm-up walking |
| 5–40 min. | Brisk walking |
| 40–45 min. | Cool-down walking |

## Duration walking plan

By increasing the duration of your walking workout, you can work on improving your overall endurance and stamina. Tables 10-7 to 10-9 outline the duration walking plan.

| Table 10-7 | Duration Walking Plan, Level 1 |
| --- | --- |
| *Time* | *Walking Type* |
| 0–5 min. | Warm-up walking |
| 5–20 min. | Moderate walking |
| 20–30 min. | Brisk walking |
| 30–35 min. | Moderate walking |
| 35–40 min. | Cool-down walking |

| Table 10-8 | Duration Walking Plan, Level 2 |
| --- | --- |
| *Time* | *Walking Type* |
| 0–5 min. | Warm-up walking |
| 5–30 min. | Moderate walking |
| 30–40 min. | Brisk walking |
| 40–50 min. | Moderate walking |
| 50–55 min. | Cool-down walking |

| Table 10-9 | Duration Walking Plan, Level 3 |
|---|---|
| **Time** | **Walking Type** |
| 0–5 min. | Warm-up walking |
| 5–30 min. | Moderate walking |
| 30–45 min. | Brisk walking |
| 45–55 min. | Moderate walking |
| 55–60 min. | Cool-down walking |

## Stress walking plan

The stress walking plan incorporates various walking speeds and breathing exercises to help you reduce your stress levels and improve your overall health. Tables 10-10 to 10-12 outline the stress walking plan.

| Table 10-10 | Stress Walking Plan, Level 1 |
|---|---|
| **Time** | **Walking Type** |
| 0–5 min. | Warm-up walking |
| 5–10 min. | Casual walking with deep breathing |
| 10–20 min. | Moderate walking |
| 20–25 min. | Casual walking with deep breathing |
| 25–30 min. | Brisk walking |
| 30–35 min. | Moderate walking |
| 35–40 min. | Cool-down walking |

| Table 10-11 | Stress Walking Plan, Level 2 |
|---|---|
| **Time** | **Walking Type** |
| 0–5 min. | Warm-up walking |
| 5–10 min. | Casual walking with deep breathing |
| 10–20 min. | Moderate walking |
| 20–21 min. | Fast walking |
| 21–25 min. | Moderate walking |
| 25–26 min. | Fast walking |

| Time | Walking Type |
|------|--------------|
| 26–30 min. | Moderate walking |
| 30–35 min. | Casual walking with deep breathing |
| 35–40 min. | Cool-down walking |

| Table 10-12 | Stress Walking Plan, Level 3 |
|-------------|------------------------------|
| Time | Walking Type |
| 0–5 min. | Warm-up walking |
| 5–10 min. | Casual walking with deep breathing |
| 10–15 min. | Brisk walking |
| 15–20 min. | Casual walking with deep breathing |
| 20–21 min. | Moderate walking |
| 21–22 min. | Fast walking |
| 22–23 min. | Moderate walking |
| 23–24 min. | Fast walking |
| 24–25 min. | Moderate walking |
| 25–26 min. | Fast walking |
| 26–27 min. | Moderate walking |
| 27–28 min. | Fast walking |
| 28–29 min. | Moderate walking |
| 29–30 min. | Fast walking |
| 30–35 min. | Casual walking with deep breathing |
| 35–40 min. | Cool-down walking |

# Resistance walking plan

The resistance walking plan, outlined in Tables 10-13 to 10-15, helps you tone and build lean body mass, or muscle mass. Muscle mass is a metabolically active tissue. By having more muscle, not only do you look more toned, but you actually boost your metabolism, burning more fat and calories.

| Table 10-13 | Resistance Walking Plan, Level 1 |
|---|---|
| *Time* | *Walking Type* |
| 0–5 min. | Warm-up walking |
| 5–10 min. | Moderate walking |
| 10–10:30 min. | Overhead shoulder press |
| 10:30–11:30 min. | Moderate walking |
| 11:30–12 min. | Lunges |
| 12–13 min. | Moderate walking |
| 13–13:30 min. | Ab squeeze |
| 13:30–14:30 min. | Brisk walking |
| 14:30–15 min. | Chest press |
| 15–16 min. | Moderate walking |
| 16–16:30 min. | Tippy-toe walking |
| 16:30–17:30 min. | Moderate walking |
| 17:30–18 min. | Triceps extensions |
| 18–19 min. | Moderate walking |
| 19–19:30 min. | Ab twists |
| 19:30–25 min. | Brisk walking |
| 25–30 min. | Cool-down walking |

| Table 10-14 | Resistance Walking Plan, Level 2 |
|---|---|
| *Time* | *Walking Type* |
| 0–5 min. | Warm-up walking |
| 5–10 min. | Moderate walking |
| 10–10:45 min. | Overhead shoulder press |
| 10:45–11:45 min. | Moderate walking |
| 11:45–12:30 min. | Lunges |
| 12:30–13:30 min. | Moderate walking |
| 13:30–14:15 min. | Ab squeeze |
| 14:15–15:15 min. | Brisk walking |

| Time | Walking Type |
|------|-------------|
| 15:15–16 min. | Chest press |
| 16–17 min. | Moderate walking |
| 17–17:45 min. | Tippy-toe walking |
| 17:45–18:45 min. | Moderate walking |
| 18:45–19:30 min. | Triceps extensions |
| 19:30–20:30 min. | Moderate walking |
| 20:30–21:15 min. | Ab twists |
| 21:15–30 min. | Brisk walking |
| 30–35 min. | Cool-down walking |

| Table 10-15 | Resistance Walking Plan, Level 3 |
|-------------|----------------------------------|
| **Time** | **Walking Type** |
| 0–5 min. | Warm-up walking |
| 5–10 min. | Moderate walking |
| 10–11 min. | Overhead shoulder press |
| 11–12 min. | Moderate walking |
| 12–13 min. | Lunges |
| 13–14 min. | Moderate walking |
| 14–15 min. | Ab squeeze |
| 15–25 min. | Brisk walking |
| 25–26 min. | Chest press |
| 26–27 min. | Moderate walking |
| 27–28 min. | Tippy-toe walking |
| 28–29 min. | Moderate walking |
| 29–30 min. | Triceps extensions |
| 30–31 min. | Moderate walking |
| 31–32 min. | Ab twists |
| 32–40 min. | Brisk walking |
| 40–45 min. | Cool-down walking |

As you look at the resistance walking plan outline, you'll notice that it calls for various exercises to be incorporated into your walk. Here's a look at each exercise and how to perform it:

- ✔ **Overhead shoulder press:** Refer to Figure 10-2. As you walk, raise both arms above your head with your elbows bent. Your hands should be beside your ears. Slowly straighten your elbows to raise your arms above your head; then return to the starting position. Perform the exercise slowly to feel the muscles working and continue to repeat the press for the duration of the time listed.

- ✔ **Chest press:** See Figure 10-3. As you walk, raise your arms up to your sides with your elbows bent and hugging your midsection. Your palms should be facing down. Slowly straighten your elbows to straighten your arms out in front of you; then return to the starting position and continue to repeat the press for the duration of the time listed.

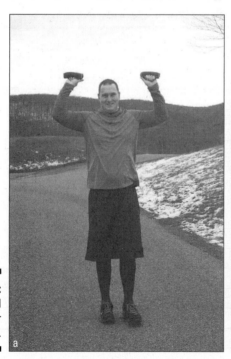 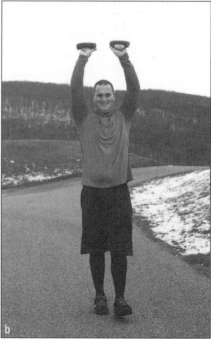

**Figure 10-2:**
Overhead
shoulder
press.

*Photos by Kristen Rath Photography*

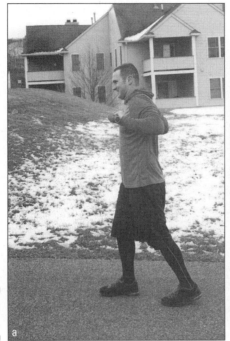 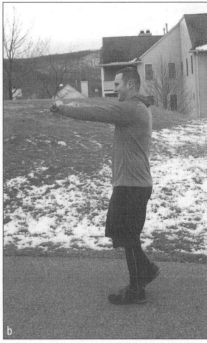

**Figure 10-3:**
Chest press.

a                                                   b

*Photos by Kristen Rath Photography*

✔ **Triceps extensions:** Refer to Figure 10-4. As you walk, take turns raising one arm above your head. With the arm straight above you, bend your elbow so that your hand is lowered back towards your bicep. Slowly straighten your elbow to raise your arm. At the top of the exercise, squeeze your triceps muscle; then repeat on the other arm. Continue this movement, alternating arms, for the duration of the time listed.

✔ **Lunges:** Take a look at Figure 10-5. As you walk, slow down your pace. Stand with good posture with your arms by your sides or your hands on your hips. Take a large step forward with one leg while lifting up onto the ball of your foot with your back leg. As you do this, keep your chest lifted and your shoulders back. Your hips should be lowering to the ground but not moving forward. Watch that your knee does not pass over your toe and that your back knee does not touch the ground. Now, press up with your front leg and bring your back leg forward. Repeat this lunge on the opposite leg. Continue to repeat one leg after the other.

✔ **Tippy-toe walking:** See Figure 10-6. Slow down your walking speed. Raise your heels up so that you are walking on the ball of your foot. Slowly walk on the balls of your feet for the listed time frame; then slowly lower your heels back down to the floor.

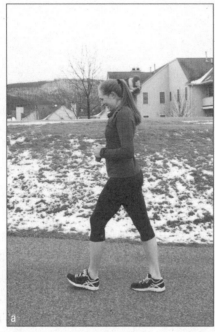 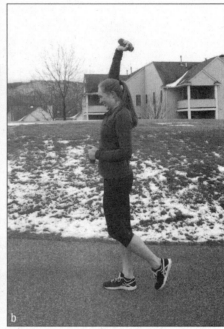

**Figure 10-4:**
Triceps
extensions.

a

b

*Photos by Kristen Rath Photography*

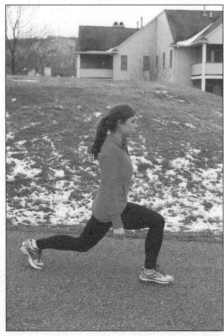

**Figure 10-5:**
Lunges.

*Photo by Kristen Rath Photography*

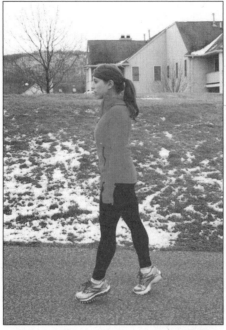

**Figure 10-6:**
Tippy-toe
walking.

*Photo by Kristen Rath Photography*

✔ **Ab squeeze:** Refer to Figure 10-7. As you are walking, think of pulling your belly button in toward your spine. As you draw your abdominals in, squeeze your ab muscles as hard as you can, activating your whole core. Continue to breathe normally as you do this. Keep your core tight and walk with your core tight and pulled in for the listed timeframe; then relax and repeat.

✔ **Ab twists:** See Figure 10-8. Perform the same movement as the ab squeeze; however, once your core is tight and your abdominals are pulled in, bring your arms to your side with your elbows bent. Slowly twist at your waist using only your core muscles and not your arms. Twist slightly to the right and then slightly to the left. You should feel your oblique muscles activating as you do this. Continue this movement for the listed period of time.

## Total body workout walking plan

Similar to the resistance walking plan, the total body workout walking plan builds and tones muscles and boosts metabolism. But whereas the resistance walking plan incorporates muscle-building exercises into the duration of your walk, the total body workout is done after the completion of your walk. Tables 10-16 to 10-18 outline the total body workout walking plan.

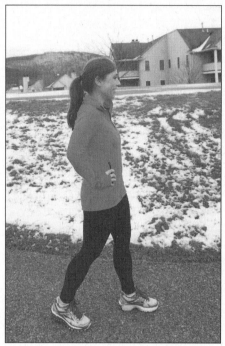

**Figure 10-7:**
Ab squeeze.

*Photo by Kristen Rath Photography*

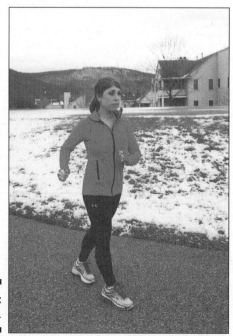

**Figure 10-8:**
Ab twists.

*Photo by Kristen Rath Photography*

| Table 10-16 | Total Body Workout Walking Plan, Level 1 |
| --- | --- |
| *Time* | *Walking Type* |
| 0–5 min. | Warm-up walking |
| 5–15 min. | Moderate walking |
| 15–20 min. | Brisk walking |
| 20–25 min. | Moderate walking |
| 25–30 min. | Cool-down walking |
| *Legs* | *Reps* |
| Calf raises | 6–8 reps |
| Hamstring curls | 6–8 reps |
| Squats | 6–8 reps |
| Glute bridge | 6–8 reps |
| *Core* | *Time/Reps* |
| Plank | 15 seconds |
| Side plank | 15 seconds |
| Swingin' abs | 6–8 reps |
| *Arms/Back* | *Reps* |
| Bicep curls | 6–8 reps |
| Triceps extensions | 6–8 reps |
| Chest presses | 6–8 reps |
| Shoulder presses | 6–8 reps |

| Table 10-17 | Total Body Workout Walking Plan, Level 2 |
| --- | --- |
| *Time* | *Walking Type* |
| 0–5 min. | Warm-up walking |
| 5–10 min. | Moderate walking |
| 10–20 min. | Brisk walking |
| 20–25 min. | Moderate walking |
| 25–30 min. | Cool-down walking |
| *Legs* | *Reps* |
| Calf raises | 8–12 reps |
| Hamstring curls | 8–12 reps |
| Squats | 8–12 reps |

*(continued)*

**Table 10-17** *(continued)*

| Legs | Reps |
| --- | --- |
| Glute bridge | 8–12 reps |
| **Core** | **Time/Reps** |
| Plank | 30 seconds |
| Side plank | 30 seconds |
| Swingin' Abs | 8–12 reps |
| **Arms/Back** | **Reps** |
| Biceps curls | 8–12 reps |
| Triceps extensions | 8–12 reps |
| Chest presses | 8–12 reps |
| Shoulder presses | 8–12 reps |

**Table 10-18    Total Body Workout Walking Plan, Level 3**

| Time | Walking Type |
| --- | --- |
| 0–5 min. | Warm-up walking |
| 5–10 min. | Moderate walking |
| 10–20 min. | Brisk walking |
| 20–25 min. | Moderate walking |
| 25–30 min. | Cool-down walking |
| **Legs** | **Reps** |
| Calf raises | 12–15 reps |
| Hamstring curls | 12–15 reps |
| Squats | 12–15 reps |
| Glute bridge | 12–15 reps |
| **Core** | **Time/Reps** |
| Plank | 45 seconds |
| Side plank | 45 seconds |
| Swingin' abs | 12–15 reps |
| **Arms/Back** | **Reps** |
| Biceps curls | 12–15 reps |
| Triceps extensions | 12–15 reps |
| Chest presses | 12–15 reps |
| Shoulder presses | 12–15 reps |

The total body workout calls for resistance exercises to be performed after completing a walk. Here's a closer look at each exercise and how it is performed:

- ✔ **Calf raises:** Refer to Figure 10-9. Stand with your feet shoulder width apart. Your feet should be firmly on the ground and your abdominals pulled in. Slowly raise your heels, lifting yourself up onto the ball of your foot. Hold this position for a moment and then lower back down. You can increase the intensity of this exercise by performing it on the edge of a step with your heels hanging over the edge or by holding light weights as you perform the exercise

- ✔ **Hamstring curls:** See Figure 10-10. Stand facing the back of a sturdy object such as a chair with your feet underneath your hips. Shift your weight onto your left leg; then slowly bend your right leg and raise your right heel up to your backside. Hold this position at the top of the curl and feel a squeeze in your hamstring; then slowly lower your leg back to the floor. Repeat on the opposite leg.

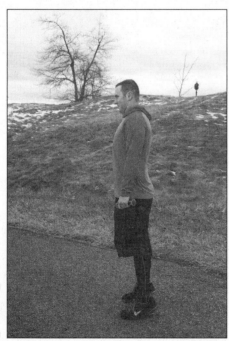

**Figure 10-9:**
Calf raises.

*Photo by Kristen Rath Photography*

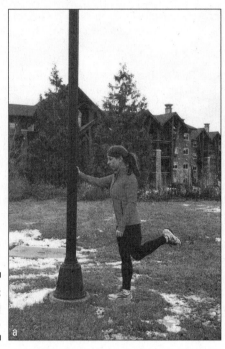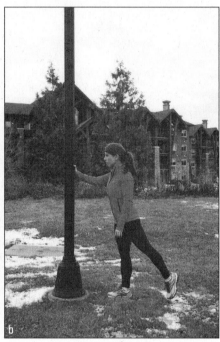

**Figure 10-10:** Hamstring curls.

*Photos by Kristen Rath Photography*

✔ **Squats:** Take a look at Figure 10-11. Stand with your feet shoulder width apart, straightening your knees and pulling in your abdominals. Bend your knees while maintaining good posture and a straight back. Deepen your knee bend until your buttocks become parallel with your knees. As you lower into your squat, make sure that your knees do not pass over your toes. Slowly straighten your knees back up to a fully upright position; then repeat.

✔ **Glute bridge:** Consult Figure 10-12. Lie down on the floor face up with your knees bent and your feet flat on the floor. Keep your arms at your sides with your palms facing down toward the floor. Raise your hips up into the air so your body creates a straight line from your knees to your shoulders. Hold this position; then lower your back slowly back down to the floor.

✔ **Plank:** Refer to Figure 10-13. Start in a basic plank position by having your hands and toes on the floor and your body outstretched. Your midsection should be straight — no arching or sagging of your back, and no sticking your butt in the air! You should be one straight line from your nose to your toes. Concentrate on keeping your core tight. Hold this position for the time listed; then relax.

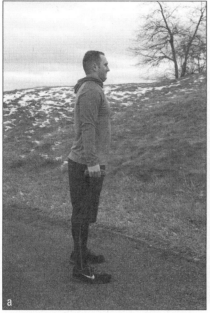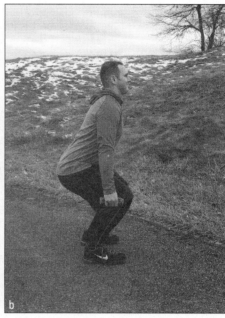

**Figure 10-11:** Squats.

a                                       b

*Photos by Kristen Rath Photography*

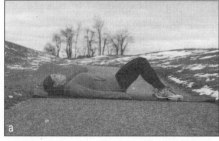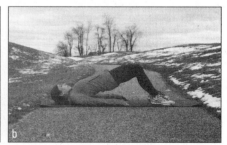

**Figure 10-12:** Glute bridge.

a                                       b

*Photos by Kristen Rath Photography*

✔ **Side plank:** See Figure 10-14. Start in the basic plank position (see the preceding bullet). Raise your right hand up to the ceiling and slightly turn your body so your right hip and side are now facing the ceiling. Don't allow your body or left hip to sag. Push your left hip toward the ceiling to keep your body in a straight line. Hold for the listed time period; then return to the basic plank position and repeat on the other side.

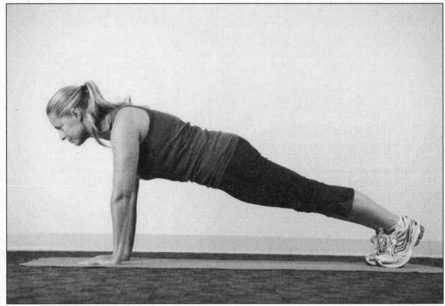

**Figure 10-13:**
Plank.

*Photo by Matt Bowen*

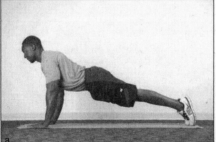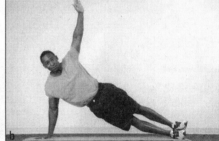

**Figure 10-14:**
Side plank.

*Photo by Matt Bowen*

✔ **Swingin' abs:** Take a look at Figure 10-15. Using a chair, stand perpendicular to the chair with your legs slightly spread at shoulder width apart (your left side should be toward the chair). Place your left hand on the chair. While keeping your core tight (pull your belly button into your spine), lift your right leg straight in front of you to hip level. In a controlled swing, lower your right leg down to the front; then swing it to the right, bringing it up straight out to your right side at hip level. Then swing your leg back in a controlled motion, first down to the front and then up to the left at hip level. Keep your core tight and your back straight as you complete this exercise. Repeat for the number of repetitions listed; then turn to the right and repeat with the left leg.

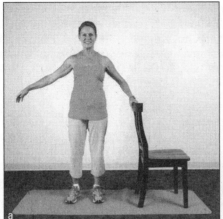
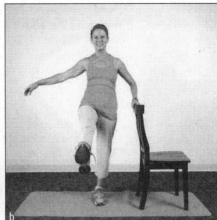
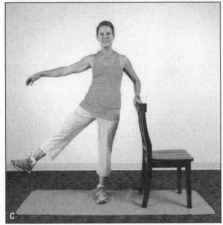

**Figure 10-15:**
Swingin'
abs.

*Photos by Matt Bowen*

- **Bicep curls:** See Figure 10-16. Stand with your feet shoulder width apart and your arms at your sides with your palms facing up. Create a fist with your hands; then slowly bend at your elbows and raise your fists up toward your shoulders. You should feel a squeeze in your biceps as you do this. At the top of the move, hold and squeeze your biceps, then slowly lower back down to the starting position. You may add resistance bands or dumbbells if you want to increase the intensity of the exercise.

- **Triceps extensions:** Stand with your feet shoulder width apart. Raise your arms straight above your head and interlock your hands. With your elbows in and perpendicular to the floor, lower your hands back toward your upper back. As you lower your hands, your upper arms should stay stationary — only your forearms should be moving. Slowly raise your forearms back to the starting position. As you reach the top, squeeze your triceps muscles; then repeat the exercise.

✔ **Chest presses:** Check out Figure 10-17. Lie down on the floor or on an incline bench with your knees bent and your feet flat on the floor. Your elbows should be bent and hugging your sides. Your palms should be facing out toward the ceiling. Slowly extend your arms by straightening your elbows; then return back to the starting position.

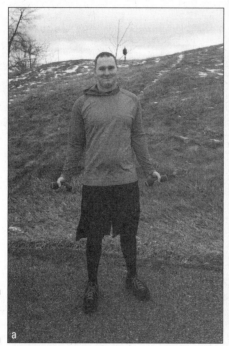
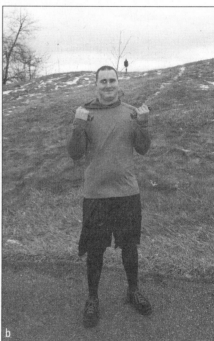

**Figure 10-16:** Bicep curls.

*Photos by Kristen Rath Photography*

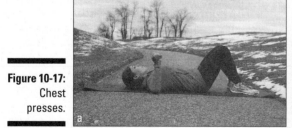
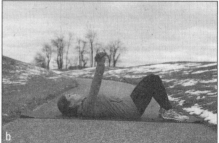

**Figure 10-17:** Chest presses.

*Photos by Kristen Rath Photography*

✔ **Shoulder presses:** Refer to Figure 10-18. Stand with your feet shoulder width apart. Your arms should be raised with your elbows bent and your palms facing out and near your ears. Straighten your elbows to raise your palms into the air; then slowly bend your elbows to return to the starting position.

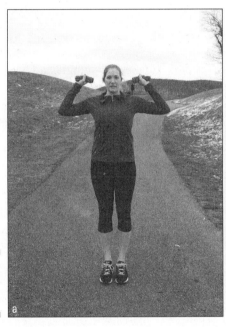 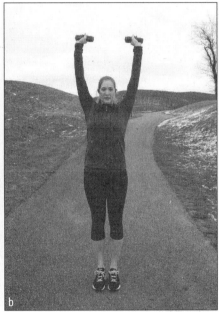

**Figure 10-18:** Shoulder presses.

*Photos by Kristen Rath Photography*

# The Walking Programs That Gear the Plans Toward Your Goal

Up to this point in the chapter, you've matched your goals with a particular program and reviewed the plans that the programs rely on to meet specific goals. Now it's time to put those plans into action by working your chosen program!

In this section I give you the lowdown on the specifics of each program. Find the program that best meets your personal goals, and follow that program's guidelines to turn your goals into reality.

You can find the details about all the plans listed in the second column of the upcoming program tables in the previous section, "The Walking Plans That Make Up the Programs." You may find using a stopwatch or timer helpful as you begin implementing your plans each day. On resting and stretching days, please refer to Chapter 6 for the best types of stretches to implement and how to perform each.

## Weight-loss maximizer program

To get started shedding the maximum number of pounds and inches, jump into the weight-loss maximizer program outlined in Table 10-19.

| Table 10-19 | Weight-Loss Maximizer Program |
| --- | --- |
| *Weeks 1 and 2* | |
| *Day* | *Plan* |
| Day 1 | Interval walking, Level 1 |
| Day 2 | Duration walking, Level 1 |
| Day 3 | Total body workout walking, Level 1 |
| Day 4 | Duration walking, Level 1 |
| Day 5 | Interval walking, Level 1 |
| Day 6 | Total body workout walking, Level 1 |
| Day 7 | Rest day or Stress walking, Level 1 |
| *Weeks 3 and 4* | |
| *Day* | *Plan* |
| Day 1 | Interval walking, Level 2 |
| Day 2 | Total body workout walk, Level 2 |
| Day 3 | Duration walking, Level 2 |
| Day 4 | Stress walking, Level 2 |
| Day 5 | Total body workout walking, Level 2 |
| Day 6 | Interval walking, Level 2 |
| Day 7 | Rest and stretch |
| *Weeks 5 and 6* | |
| *Day* | *Plan* |
| Day 1 | Total body workout walking, Level 3 |
| Day 2 | Duration walking, Level 3 |

| Weeks 5 and 6 | |
|---|---|
| **Day** | **Plan** |
| Day 3 | Interval walking, Level 3 |
| Day 4 | Duration walking, Level 3 |
| Day 5 | Total body workout walking, Level 3 |
| Day 6 | Interval walking, Level 3 |
| Day 7 | Rest day or stress walking, Level 3 |

# Fitness enhancer program

If you are serious about increasing your strength, endurance, and speed, then the fitness enhancer program is the one for you. See Table 10-20 for an outline of the program.

| Table 10-20 | Fitness Enhancer Program |
|---|---|
| **Weeks 1 and 2** | |
| **Day** | **Plan** |
| Day 1 | Duration walking, Level 1 |
| Day 2 | Interval walking, Level 1 |
| Day 3 | Resistance walking, Level 1 |
| Day 4 | Speed walking, Level 1 |
| Day 5 | Interval walking, Level 1 |
| Day 6 | Duration walking, Level 1 |
| Day 7 | Rest and stretch |
| **Weeks 3 and 4** | |
| **Day** | **Plan** |
| Day 1 | Speed walking, Level 2 |
| Day 2 | Total body workout walking, Level 1 |
| Day 3 | Duration walking, Level 2 |
| Day 4 | Interval walking, Level 2 |
| Day 5 | Resistance walking, Level 2 |
| Day 6 | Speed walking, Level 2 |
| Day 7 | Rest and stretch |

*(continued)*

**Table 10-20** *(continued)*

| *Weeks 5 and 6* | |
| --- | --- |
| *Day* | *Plan* |
| Day 1 | Duration walking, Level 3 |
| Day 2 | Interval walking, Level 3 |
| Day 3 | Speed walking, Level 3 |
| Day 4 | Total body workout walking, Level 2 |
| Day 5 | Duration walking, Level 3 |
| Day 6 | Interval walking, Level 3 |
| Day 7 | Rest and stretch |

# Stress buster program

If you need to reduce stress to improve your overall health and shed pounds, then the stress buster program is perfect for you. Table 10-21 outlines the full program.

| **Table 10-21** | **Stress Buster Program** |
| --- | --- |
| *Weeks 1 and 2* | |
| *Day* | *Plan* |
| Day 1 | Stress walking, Level 1 |
| Day 2 | Duration walking, Level 1 |
| Day 3 | Stress walking, Level 1 |
| Day 4 | Resistance walking, Level 1 |
| Day 5 | Stress walking, Level 1 |
| Day 6 | Interval walking, Level 1 |
| Day 7 | Stress walking, Level 1 |
| *Weeks 3 and 4* | |
| *Day* | *Plan* |
| Day 1 | Stress walking, Level 2 |
| Day 2 | Duration walking, Level 2 |

| Weeks 3 and 4 | |
|---|---|
| **Day** | **Plan** |
| Day 3 | Stress walking, Level 2 |
| Day 4 | Resistance walking, Level 2 |
| Day 5 | Stress walking, Level 2 |
| Day 6 | Interval walking, Level 2 |
| Day 7 | Stress walking, Level 2 |
| **Weeks 5 and 6** | |
| **Day** | **Plans** |
| Day 1 | Stress walking, Level 3 |
| Day 2 | Duration walking, Level 3 |
| Day 3 | Stress walking, Level 3 |
| Day 4 | Resistance walking, Level 3 |
| Day 5 | Stress walking, Level 3 |
| Day 6 | Interval walking, Level 3 |
| Day 7 | Stress walking, Level 3 |

# Disease fighter program

If you need to start getting serious about your health, the disease fighter program is the right choice! This walking program helps you shed pounds and inches while lowering blood pressure, cholesterol, and blood sugar levels. See Table 10-22 for the full program.

| Table 10-22 | Disease Fighter Program |
|---|---|
| **Weeks 1 and 2** | |
| **Day** | **Plan** |
| Day 1 | Duration walking, Level 1 |
| Day 2 | Interval walking, Level 1 |
| Day 3 | Resistance walking, Level 1 |
| Day 4 | Stress walking, Level 1 |
| Day 5 | Duration walking, Level 1 |
| Day 6 | Stress walking, Level 1 |
| Day 7 | Rest and stretch |

*(continued)*

### Table 10-22 *(continued)*

#### Weeks 3 and 4

| Day | Plan |
| --- | --- |
| Day 1 | Total body workout walking, Level 1 |
| Day 2 | Duration walking, Level 2 |
| Day 3 | Interval walking, Level 2 |
| Day 4 | Stress walking, Level 2 |
| Day 5 | Total body workout walking, Level 1 |
| Day 6 | Duration walking, Level 2 |
| Day 7 | Stretch and/or stress walking, Level 2 |

#### Weeks 5 and 6

| Day | Plan |
| --- | --- |
| Day 1 | Stress walking, Level 3 |
| Day 2 | Interval walking, Level 3 |
| Day 3 | Resistance walking, Level 2 |
| Day 4 | Stress walking, Level 3 |
| Day 5 | Duration walking Level 3 |
| Day 6 | Stress walking, Level 3 |
| Day 7 | Rest and stretch |

## Managing menopause program

If menopause has you seeing the scale increase and your waistline expand, don't panic. This program will have you back in your skinny jeans in no time. See Table 10-23 for the full program.

## Boosting daily activity program

If you want to start walking to improve your overall health and drop unwanted pounds, but are not able to or don't have the time to fit in scheduled exercise to your day, then this is the plan for you. Using a pedometer, you can slowly increase your overall daily steps each week until you achieve the desired activity level for optimal health and body weight. See Table 10-24 for the program details.

| Table 10-23 | Managing Menopause Program |
|---|---|
| *Weeks 1 and 2* | |
| *Day* | *Workout* |
| Day 1 | Total body workout walking, Level 1 |
| Day 2 | Interval walking, Level 1 |
| Day 3 | Stress walking, Level 1 |
| Day 4 | Total body workout walking, Level 1 |
| Day 5 | Interval walking, Level 1 |
| Day 6 | Speed walking, Level 1 |
| Day 7 | Rest and stretch |
| *Weeks 3 and 4* | |
| *Day* | *Workout* |
| Day 1 | Speed walking, Level 2 |
| Day 2 | Total body workout walking, Level 2 |
| Day 3 | Interval walking, Level 2 |
| Day 4 | Duration walking, Level 2 |
| Day 5 | Total body workout walking, Level 2 |
| Day 6 | Interval walking, Level 2 |
| Day 7 | Stress walking, Level 2, or rest and stretch |
| *Weeks 5 and 6* | |
| *Day* | *Workout* |
| Day 1 | Total body workout walking, Level 3 |
| Day 2 | Interval walking, Level 3 |
| Day 3 | Stress walking, Level 3 |
| Day 4 | Total body workout walking, Level 3 |
| Day 5 | Interval walking, Level 3 |
| Day 6 | Speed walking, Level 3 |
| Day 7 | Rest and stretch |

| Table 10-24 | Boosting Daily Activity Program |
|---|---|
| **Week** | **Goal** |
| Week 1 | Wear a pedometer from the moment you wake up until you go to bed every day this week. After seven days, take the average of the number of steps you walked each day. |
| Week 2 | Increase your daily steps by 500 above your average number each day this week. |
| Week 3 | Increase your daily steps by 1,500 above your average number each day this week. |
| Week 4 | Increase your daily steps by 2,500 above your average number each day this week. |
| Week 5 | Increase your daily steps by 3,500 above your average number each day this week. |
| Week 6 | Aim to walk a minimum of 10,000 steps everyday or at least 4,000 steps more than your original average number of steps (whichever is greater). |

# Chapter 11

# Taking Your Workout to the Next Level

*In This Chapter*

▶ Determining when you need to adjust your walking workout

▶ Burning more calories while you walk

▶ Adding strength training to your workout

▶ Dealing with plateaus

*Y*ou've started your walking workout and the pounds and inches have been coming off. You're loving your results, but now you want more. Maybe you feel that your workout isn't challenging your fitness in the same way it once was. Or maybe you feel as though your rate of weight loss is slowing a bit. When it comes to exercise, the more you do it, the more fit you become. And while this is great for your health, it can have a less than ideal impact on weight loss.

As your fitness level increases, your walking workout becomes less challenging to your body. Although this means your heart and muscles have become stronger, it also means you burn fewer calories during your workout than you once did. The walking workouts in this book are customized to change every two weeks and evolve to continue to challenge your body and maximize the amount of calories you burn. However, after completing six weeks of your walking workout and mastering Level 3 of your routine, you may be looking for ways to continue to challenge yourself and see results at the same pace.

Completing Level 3 of your walking workout doesn't mean that you necessarily need to increase the intensity of your workout right away. People differ as to when they need to change their individual workout routine to continue to see results. If you're continuing to lose at least 1/2 to 2 pounds of weight per week (if you haven't already achieved your weight-loss goal), then your plan is still working great for you and there's no need to adjust it yet. However, when your weight loss begins to slow and you're still a ways away from your ultimate goal, a change may be needed.

# Knowing When to Adjust Your Walking Routine

As I'm sure you know, everyone who wants to lose weight would like to do so instantly. And it would be wonderful if that was possible, but it isn't. That doesn't mean you can't reach your ultimate goals, but it does take patience and time. You also have to be realistic about the progress you're making when it comes to your walking workout so you know if and when you need to make adjustments. Losing weight at the rate of 1/2 pound to 2 pounds per week is normal progress. If your weight loss slows to less than half a pound per week, you may want to consider making changes to your workout.

However, keep in mind that one week at the same weight does not equal a weight-loss plateau. Your body isn't a machine and doesn't lose weight at the exact same rate from week to week. Look at your weight-loss average after completing the six-week course outlined in this book. What was your average rate of weight loss per week? If you averaged 1 pound per week, unless your rate of weight loss falls far below this or stalls for a period of a few weeks, you don't need to adjust your weight loss plan just yet.

So how do you know when it's time to make an adjustment to your walking workout? Here are the signs to be on the lookout for:

✔ Your workout no longer feels like a workout; it seems too easy.

✔ Your heart rate doesn't reach your target zone.

✔ Your weight hasn't changed for three weeks or more.

✔ You haven't seen an increase in inches lost in over a month.

✔ You no longer feel as though your strength and/or endurance are increasing.

If you're experiencing at least one of the preceding signs (and you have not already reached your goal weight or goal waist circumference), it may be time to change your walking workout to speed up your results.

# Maximizing the Calorie Burn of Your Walking Workout

In order to lose weight or shed inches faster, you need to challenge your body to burn more calories. To do this, you can either exercise longer or harder.

If increasing the intensity of your walking workout feels too challenging or isn't something you want to tackle right now, you can always increase the length or duration of your walk. For instance, walking an extra mile per day may result in losing another pound per month. Or adding an extra ten minutes to your walking workout may increase the rate at which you shrink your waistline.

However, walking farther or longer isn't always practical. One of the main reasons people get off track with exercise is that they struggle to find the time to fit it in. Increasing the length of your workout may only make fitting your walk into your day more challenging. And the last thing you want to do is start giving yourself a reason to exercise less! Instead, you can maximize the amount of calories you burn per minute by simply changing your walking routine. You can do this in a number of ways. Throughout this chapter, I show you techniques you can use to increase the rate of calories you burn during your walking workout; you can decide which one works best for you.

There are three main ways to go about increasing the intensity of your workout and the number of calories that you burn:

- ✔ Adding incline
- ✔ Adding speed
- ✔ Adding resistance

Adding one of these options is a surefire way to boost your walking workout; however, you can choose to add two or even all three to your workout to really step things up.

When intensifying your workout, you should make sure to do it gradually over time to protect against injury as well as prevent burnout. As I show you these techniques in detail, I help you to see how you can begin to add each into your workout gradually to protect your body while continuing to see results.

## Adding an incline to impact your workout

Think of the last time you climbed up a large flight of stairs. Did you feel a little winded at the top? Did you feel like climbing the stairs was more of a workout then walking on a flat surface? Most likely your answer to both of these questions is "yes." That's because adding an incline to your walk challenges your body and your muscles in a different way. Walking uphill makes the muscles in your legs — including your calves, hamstrings, and glutes — work harder. The harder your muscles work, the more energy they burn.

And burning more energy means burning more fat and calories. And the more calories you burn, the faster you'll see that weight-loss result you're after. You can go about adding an incline in a few ways:

- ✔ **Choose hilly terrain:** If you're walking outside, change your walking route to one that includes hills.

- ✔ **Adjust the incline:** If you're walking on a treadmill, use a treadmill that allows you to adjust the incline level, and do so gradually.

- ✔ **March:** If neither hills nor an incline are available, you can simulate walking on an incline by walking with "high knees" — kicking your knees up as though you're marching when you walk.

- ✔ **Incorporate stairs:** You may also choose to walk up and down a stairway in your home or in a public location (such as a shopping mall) for part of your walk to increase the intensity of your walk.

## Increasing your speed and intensity

Increasing the speed and intensity of your walking workout is a sure way to boost your calorie burn. But you also have to be realistic when you make changes to your workout. Going from a leisurely pace to speed walking can be quite an adjustment. A higher-intensity workout places a bit more wear and tear on your body. It can also be more taxing mentally as well as physically. If you push yourself too hard, you can go from feeling energized after your workout and looking forward to the next one to feeling exhausted and dreading your next workout.

Remember, in order to see weight-loss results — and keep them — you need to be consistent with your walking workout. A less-intense workout that you do daily is more beneficial to long-term weight loss and health than a very intense workout that you only do once or twice a week. Not only do you want to avoid burning yourself out, but you also want to protect yourself against injury. If you push too hard and too fast, you can injure yourself and end up sidelined instead of being able to workout.

If you decide to add an incline to your workout or boost your speed to increase your calorie burn, do so gradually. For instance, if you're walking on a treadmill that has an incline, raise it only 1 to 2 percent and walk at that incline for a week. Then increase the incline once that level feels easy or comfortable, which may happen after a week or two. Use the same strategy if you increase your speed. If you're walking at a level at which you can comfortably carry on a conversation, pick up the pace to a level at which you can still speak a sentence at a time, but can't have a full conversation. You don't want to walk so fast that you can barely speak, because at that point your heart rate is too high, and challenging your body that much physically can be dangerous.

# Interval training

Throughout this book I mention that interval training, where you repeatedly walk at a slower speed for a few minutes and then walk as quickly as you can for a set period of time, can maximize your weight-loss results. In Chapter 10, you see that many of the walking programs incorporate the Interval Walking Plan to challenge you and shed pounds and inches. But, you may be wondering why and how interval training works.

If you want to lose weight faster and burn more calories without increasing the time that you spend walking, interval training may be just what you're looking for. This form of training, which was once used only by high-level athletes, has benefits for the everyday exerciser as well. Although it may sound complicated, it's really pretty simple. Interval training is just alternating lower-intensity exercise with bursts of high-intensity exercise. When it comes to walking, interval training is essentially alternating between walking at a slower speed for a few minutes and walking at a much faster pace for a period of time. You can also incorporate interval training with incline. Instead of changing your speed, you alternate between walking on a flat surface for a period of time and walking at a high incline. Simple, right?

Incorporating interval training can offer many benefits, including the following:

- **Maximizing the calories that you burn:** Even if you add only a few short bursts of interval training into your workout, you'll burn more calories and fat, helping you to see results faster.

- **Preventing your workout from becoming mundane:** If walking the same route over and over is causing you to become bored with your workout, spicing it up by adding intervals can keep it interesting and help you to stay motivated.

- **Increasing your cardiovascular fitness:** Interval training helps you increase your endurance faster. Better endurance means that you're able to walk longer and faster sooner than someone who doesn't incorporate interval training. Not only does this help you to achieve your weight goals more quickly, but it also helps you improve your health faster.

As you can see, there are many benefits from incorporating interval training into your walking workout. You may, however, be wondering whether interval training is right for you. If you have a chronic health condition or have not exercised before, speak with your doctor first. Recent research indicates that this type of training may be safe even for individuals with heart disease, if done for only short periods of time and eased into gradually. As with any exercise, it's always important to speak to your health care provider before starting or changing an exercise routine. Interval training may be a great option for you, but even if you are in terrific health, listen to your body. Ease into interval training slowly. Follow the guidelines in the walking programs listed in Chapter 10.

Doing too much too soon won't lead to faster results. Instead, it may lead to injury and sideline your ability to reach your long-term goals.

# Increasing Strength While Walking

When you think about walking, you may not think of building muscle, but you can actually strengthen muscle with your walking workout. When you aim to lose weight, you want to focus on ways to boost your metabolism. Your *metabolism* is the number of calories you burn each day. The more calories you burn each day, the easier it is to lose weight and keep it off. Think about it this way: You need a deficit of 500 calories per day to lose 1 pound per week. If your metabolism burns 1,800 calories, you need to reduce your intake to just 1,300 calories per day to lose 1 pound per week. However, if you were able to burn 2,000 calories per day instead of 1,800, you could eat 1,500 calories per day and lose the same amount of weight.

Metabolism is determined by many factors including age, height, body weight, and gender. In addition, the amount of lean body mass, or muscle mass, you have impacts your metabolism. The more muscle you have, the more calories you burn each day, even when you're sleeping, which gives you an advantage when trying to lose weight. So how can you boost your metabolism? The easiest way is by increasing and maintaining your current muscle mass.

As you walk, you use the muscles in your lower body as well as your abdomen to propel you forward. However, you can engage additional muscles during your walking workout, thereby increasing muscle gains in strength and size, by adding resistance to your walking workout. Doing so incorporates the muscles of your upper body into your workout, helping you burn more calories during the workout as well as for hours afterward.

If you are looking to further challenge yourself while boosting your strength and metabolism, adding resistance to your walking workout may be for you. As you see in Chapter 10, both the Total Body Walking Plan and the Resistance Walking Plan incorporate strength-training exercises during and/or after your walking workout. These plans help to challenge all your major muscle groups while still giving you a cardiovascular workout. The combination of cardiovascular exercise with resistance training has been shown to be the most effective at shedding pounds and inches and keeping them off. In addition, this combination has been shown to be the best way to keep blood vessels and your heart young and healthy, helping in the fight against heart disease.

## Deciding when to add strength training to your walk

How do you know when it's time to add resistance to your workout? The right time can really be any time. It's never too soon or too late to start thinking of ways to tone your body and strengthen your muscles. However, you can look for some signs that may indicate it's time to start adding in strength training:

✔ Your workout starts to feel too easy. You don't really feel as though you "worked out" at the end of it.

✔ Now that you have lost some weight, you're happy to start fitting into smaller clothes, but you're not yet satisfied with your muscle tone and want to become firmer.

✔ Your muscles are adjusting. Perhaps in the beginning, the muscles in your lower body felt fatigued after a walk or even slightly sore the next day. But now you feel as though you could keep on walking at the end of your workout, and you want to challenge your muscles once again.

Strength training can be a beneficial part of your walking workout, but it may not be appropriate for everyone. If you suffer from joint pain, have arthritis or osteoporosis, or are recovering from a joint or bone injury, make sure to discuss adding strength training to your walking workout with your doctor first to see whether you may need to take any precautions. If you have heart disease or diabetes, make sure to get clearance from your healthcare provider before adding resistance training. You can reference Chapters 12 and 13 for more guidelines on exercising with these conditions.

## Choosing the techniques and tools for adding resistance

When it comes to adding resistance into your walking workout, you have many options. You can

✔ Incorporate resistance as you walk

✔ Incorporate resistance after completing your walk

✔ Increase the weight you carry as you walk

All of these techniques help to increase the amount of calories you burn throughout your workout as well as increase strength, stamina, and metabolism.

Chapter 10 shows you how resistance can be incorporated into or after a walk with the Total Body Workout Walking Plan and the Resistance Walking Plan. With the Resistance Walking Plan, you actually incorporate strengthening exercises while you are walking. This plan allows you to keep your heart rate elevated while incorporating muscle building exercises for a maximum calorie burn. Because you incorporate these exercises while walking, you add resistance by using your own body weight (rather than adding weights) to prevent against injury.

As you become more accustomed to exercising with the Resistance Walking Plan, you may consider using resistance bands to further increase resistance and add strength while walking.

Using dumbbells while walking isn't recommended due to the increased chance of injury as well as the technical aspect of having to carry them for the duration of your walk. With resistance bands, even if you needed to drop them, the risk of injury would be low. For instance, a 5-pound dumbbell falling on your foot would do much more damage than a featherweight resistance band.

You still need to be cautious, however, even when using resistance bands. Maintaining good form is key to preventing injury. That's why it's best to start the Resistance Walking Plan without any added resistance to gain a level of familiarity and comfort with the exercises and understand the proper form. After you have mastered these aspects, you may then consider adding resistance bands to your workout.

Unlike the Resistance Walking Plan, the Total Body Workout Walking Plan is completed after the duration of your walk. This plan allows for your heart rate to be elevated at the start of the strength-training workout, so it can be maintained at an elevated level, burning more calories. Because you do this workout after your walk, incorporating weights, such as dumbbells, is more appropriate here. You can do these exercises using your own body weight to start, but when that ceases to be challenging, you can add light weights.

Using either resistance bands or dumbbells is appropriate in this exercise plan, but just as with any strength-training program, good form is key. To protect against injury, make sure you perform each exercise slowly and with perfect form. Don't use a weight that is too heavy, or your form will suffer and your risk for injury will increase. As with the Resistance Walking Plan, make sure you understand each exercise and can do it with correct form with no weight before adding resistance.

# *Preventing Workout Plateaus*

Plateaus happen. They can be frustrating, but they don't have to derail your progress or cause you to lose motivation. In fact, if you know how to work through a plateau, you can actually use it to your advantage. When it comes to managing a walking workout plateau, you first have to determine whether you have really reached one.

A *plateau* is when your progress stalls and you are seeing no change in weight or loss of inches while following the same walking workout and eating plan that you have been following. Sometimes, you can feel like you aren't making any progress but not actually be experiencing a plateau. When you first start any weight-loss plan, such as walking to lose weight, the pounds can start to come off rapidly. This is because in addition to losing actual fat mass, your body is also shedding water weight. Once this excess water has been lost, you begin losing fat mass — the weight you want to lose. But because fat mass comes off more slowly, it can look like the scale is slowing down, and you may become frustrated and feel as though your progress has stalled.

At this point you need to be careful. After the initial water weight losses, it's normal for progress to slow. But slow progress is still progress — it's not a plateau. You may be shedding fat yet building muscle as your body gets stronger. This change can make your weight-loss progress appear to stall, but you're actually changing your overall body composition as you gain lean body mass and shed unwanted fat mass. To help you determine whether slowed or stalled weight loss on the scale may be due to increased muscle mass, it's important to monitor your body measurements. Measure your waist circumference, your hips, your bust, your upper arms, and your thighs. Track these measurements over a period of one to three weeks. If your measurements are decreasing but your weight on the scale remains the same, most likely you are losing fat and gaining muscle. In this situation, you are still making progress and there's no need to adjust your exercise or meal plan until progress stalls.

If over a period of three to four weeks you have lost no weight and seen no decrease in measurement on any part of your body, this experience can be considered stalled progress, or a plateau. When you reach a plateau, it's important to change your exercise plan, your meal plan, or a combination of both to further jumpstart your progress. Keep in mind, however, that if your progress has stalled and you are now at a healthy body weight and have an ideal waist circumference, you may indeed be at your goal weight. In that case, you just have to work on maintaining it.

## Finding the cause of the plateau

If you've been following your walking workout plan as outlined and aren't seeing any weight-loss progress, there may be a few reasons. You may be

✔ Consuming more calories than you had previously

✔ Decreasing your overall activity (steps) throughout the day

The formula for losing weight is relatively simple: You need to burn more calories than you take in. If you are increasing the amount of calories that you burn by increasing your exercise level with walking but aren't losing weight, you're most likely taking in more calories than you realize. Starting a walking workout may have increased your appetite. Perhaps you are eating larger portions at meals, or maybe you are eating an extra snack that you didn't have in the past. Even though it may not seem significant, these little extras here and there can add up.

Don't be fooled into thinking that because you're scheduling a walking workout each day, you are automatically burning more calories. Sometimes, when you start to exercise, you may find yourself sitting more the rest of the day. If you used to be up and running around the house doing chores at night and now find yourself sitting on the couch, you're burning fewer calories in the evening than you once were. Your walking workout may take you back to reaching the level of calories you were burning when you were more active overall throughout the day, but it isn't helping you to burn additional calories to shed pounds and inches.

## Breaking through a plateau

When it comes to breaking through a plateau, the more you can track what you are doing, the better. Keeping a food record of everything you eat and drink daily is the best way to truly know what you are putting into your body. Food records are so beneficial that people who keep them lose 40 percent more weight than those who don't! To keep a record, record the time you eat, everything you eat and drink (including condiments, creamer in coffee, and so on), and the portion size of everything you eat and drink. After keeping a record for a week, determine what your average calorie intake is. Try reducing this by just 100 to 200 calories per day, and you'll start to see the scale move downward once again.

If you are eating well and walking regularly, you may think you're doing everything right. But you may be decreasing your overall daily movement, causing you to burn fewer calories and stifling your progress. To avoid this, start using a pedometer. From the time you get out of bed in the morning

until the time you lie back down, wear your pedometer to track your overall daily steps. You should aim for a minimum of 10,000 steps per day. Say you used to walk 12,000 steps per day before starting your walking workout. Now, you schedule in a daily walk that provides you with 6,000 steps, but because you are mostly sedentary the rest of the day, your total daily steps are only 9,000. This change results in you burning about 150 fewer calories than you were before you even started exercising. That's why it's so important to not only exercise regularly daily, but to make sure your level of overall physical activity stays elevated to see the best results for your weight as well as your health.

# Part IV
# Walking Considerations for Any Condition

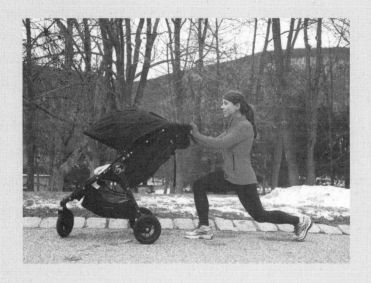

# In this part . . .

- Learn how walking can be a safe and effective way to lose weight for almost anyone.

- Discover the best ways to implement your walking workout with health conditions such as diabetes, heart disease, and arthritis.

- Understand the most common obstacles faced when working to walk off the weight, and how to best overcome them.

- Find out how to maintain your weight loss once you have achieved your goal weight.

# Chapter 12

# Walking to Improve Diabetes

## In This Chapter

▶ Determining the impact walking has on diabetes

▶ Understanding how walking can improve glucose management

▶ Seeing how walking can decrease the risk of developing diabetes

▶ Taking the necessary precautions and making the most of your workout

*O*ver 26 million Americans have diabetes; however, many are not even aware that they have the condition. As many as one in two individuals over the age of 65 have a condition known as insulin resistance or prediabetes. Could you be at risk for developing diabetes? Perhaps you have already been diagnosed. Cardiovascular health declines twice as rapidly in people with elevated glucose levels, such as those with diabetes, as compared to individuals with healthy levels. In fact, a diagnosis of diabetes makes you four times more likely to suffer a heart attack or stroke. In addition, diabetes puts you at greater risk of developing complications such as neuropathy, kidney failure, and blindness.

However, the good news is that diabetes is a preventable and manageable condition. With lifestyle changes, you can avoid developing type 2 diabetes and can manage both type 1 and type 2 diabetes effectively to help prevent and delay complications associated with the disease. Eating a healthy diet, maintaining a healthy weight, and staying physically active, such as by walking daily, are some of the best ways to improve glucose control and therefore manage diabetes.

## Understanding Diabetes

When it comes to understanding diabetes, first you have to understand the various types of this disease. Many individuals with diabetes are unaware of what type of the disease they have. Understanding what type of diabetes you have been diagnosed with is key to helping you manage the condition and improve glucose levels. Following are the various forms of diabetes:

- **Type 1:** Type 1 diabetes is an autoimmune disease where the body attacks the beta cells of the pancreas, rendering them unable to produce insulin. As the body can no longer produce its own source of insulin, external insulin is needed to live.

- **Type 2:** Type 2 diabetes is a progressive disease in which the body's cells become increasingly resistant to insulin. As cells become resistant to insulin, they disallow insulin to enter them, forcing glucose to remain in the bloodstream where it elevates over time.

- **Early insulin resistance/prediabetes:** A precursor to type 2 diabetes, prediabetes is an early stage of insulin resistance that leads to a slow increase in glucose levels. If diet and lifestyle changes are not made, this condition often progresses to type 2 diabetes. During this phase, blood glucose levels begin to rise due to insulin resistance, but are not yet high enough to be classified as having diabetes.

- **Latent autoimmune disease in adults (LADA):** This is a slow, progressive autoimmune disease where the pancreas becomes unable to produce insulin over time. Due to its gradual natural and because it's diagnosed in adulthood, this disease is often misdiagnosed as type 2 diabetes. However, over time, external insulin is needed as the pancreas continues to decrease in function.

Type 2 diabetes and prediabetes are the two forms of this disease that are most impacted by physical activity. Because these conditions are brought on by your cells becoming desensitized to insulin and therefore not allowing it to bring glucose into your cells for energy, engaging in an activity that makes your cells more sensitive to insulin is key in improving glucose control. Promoting better glucose control may help you better manage these conditions or prevent them all together.

## Can walking impact diabetes outcomes?

When you think about how many individuals are affected by diabetes and the significant and serious health problems it can cause, preventing this disease — or managing it as well as possible if you've already been diagnosed — is critical to improving longevity and quality of life. It may sound so simple, but just walking a little bit more every day can have a dramatic impact on your odds of developing diabetes or a related complication.

The most common form of diabetes, type 2 diabetes, is brought on by insulin resistance. A recent study by the University of Michigan found that when people who were considered to have prediabetes, or insulin resistance, walked one hour daily, they were able to improve their insulin sensitivity by as much as 59 percent. The participants were also found to have an improved ability to make insulin by as much as 31 percent. These results themselves are very exciting, but the time period it took to achieve these results is what makes this study remarkable! These changes in the ability to produce insulin and increase insulin sensitivity were all seen after just seven days of walking! So not only can walking play a major role in the long-term management of diabetes, but it can also greatly improve your health in as little as a few days!

Not only can walking help to improve glucose and insulin levels in those already diagnosed with diabetes, but it can also play a major role in preventing the development of the disease. One landmark study found that people who were insulin resistant were able to reduce their odds of developing type 2 diabetes by as much as 58 percent just by walking regularly. Because a diagnosis of diabetes can increase the risk of developing many health conditions such as heart disease and dementia, you can't afford not to start walking to prevent or manage this condition for a healthier — and happier — you.

To successfully manage diabetes, having the right gear is essential. Having the proper shoes, socks, and monitoring supplies are all critical to a successful walking and weight-loss routine. You can find a wide variety of these items at big box retailers like Target or specialty medical stores that have a wider selection. In addition, you can visit my website at www.erinpalinski-author.com for a current list of the best retailers (and coupons!) along with detailed comparisons of many of these products.

## Determining whether walking is right for your situation

As you can see, walking offers many wonderful benefits for individuals who are at risk of developing diabetes or already have diabetes. However, exercise in general, in almost any form, can help to improve insulin sensitivity and prevent or delay complications associated with diabetes. That's why you want to ask yourself whether walking may be the best, and most appropriate, exercise for you.

When choosing a form of exercise to prevent or manage diabetes, ask yourself a few questions to determine the best exercise for you:

✔ Is it an exercise I can do anytime or anywhere?

✔ Is it an exercise I will enjoy?

✔ Is it an exercise I can do without too much added stress on my body and without joint discomfort or pain?

✔ Is it a safe exercise for me?

Think about various forms of exercise you may want to try. Then ask yourself the preceding questions with regard to each form of exercise you identify. Can you answer "yes" to each question? If not, do you think you can realistically do this form of exercise on a regular basis?

Low-impact exercises such as swimming, biking, and walking can all offer fantastic health benefits. The biggest concern with an activity such as swimming is that you can't do it just anywhere. You have to have access to a pool, a lake, or an ocean. Swimming, if done outdoors, is also dependent on the weather. In winter, it would be hard to continue to keep up with a swimming program unless you had access to an indoor pool. Biking can be done indoors and outdoors, but you'd still have to have access to your bike when you are ready and able to exercise. If you have a stationary bike at home but decide lunchtime at work is the best time for you to exercise, you may not be able to go home, bike, and come back to work in a reasonable timeframe, limiting your ability to exercise.

Walking is not only a lower-impact exercise that offers less wear and tear on your joints and body, but it also can be done anywhere, anytime. You can walk outdoors, indoors, at work, at home, when traveling, and so on. An exercise that's not only versatile but also safe and effective is one that you will stick with. In order to gain long-term health benefits and continue to lower glucose levels and prevent or delay diabetes-related complications, it's important that you not just start getting physically active, but stay that way. Walking is your number-one choice when it comes to finding an exercise that meets all your needs, and it provides you with all the health benefits you are looking for.

# Walking to Control Glucose Levels

As I outline earlier in this chapter, walking plays a major role in preventing the development of type 2 diabetes as well as helping to reduce glucose levels in those with the condition. However, it isn't just those with type 2 diabetes who benefit from walking.

Individuals with type 1 diabetes and LADA can benefit from walking as well. Although these conditions are brought on by an immune response that prevents the body from producing its own insulin, individuals with these conditions can develop insulin resistance over time as well. Inactivity, weight gain, poor dietary choices, increased stress levels, and aging can all make someone who needs to take external insulin for survival resistant against this insulin. When this situation occurs, the affected individual has to take a higher and higher amount of insulin, which can have its own negative effects as well.

Physical activity helps to reduce and manage glucose control by making your cells more sensitive to insulin. Think about insulin as though it's a car. This car drives through your body, picks up glucose (sugar) in your bloodstream, and drives it into your cells. You can think of your cells as a garage the car needs to enter with its passenger (glucose). Now, in a healthy cell, the "garage" opens up easily and allows insulin to come right in and bring glucose along with it. However, a cell that starts to become resistant to insulin acts instead like a locked garage door. Insulin still picks up its glucose "passenger," but now the cells won't open up the "garage door" to let it in. This forces insulin back out into your bloodstream, and with it, glucose is forced back out as well. The more cells that won't let insulin in, the more glucose that builds up in your bloodstream.

Regular exercise with walking acts like a key for your body. It opens the "garage doors" in the cells back up, allowing insulin to enter once again. When insulin can enter the cells, it can bring glucose in to be used as energy, as it should be, preventing it from elevating in your bloodstream.

## Walking when glucose levels are elevated

When your glucose levels are elevated, you need to understand what has caused them to rise. Did you eat more carbohydrates than normal at your last meal or snack? Were you less physically active than normal? Are you under a large amount of stress or fighting off an illness or infection? Did you forget to take your medication or miss a dose of insulin? Once you understand why your glucose levels are elevated, you can work to prevent it from happening in the future. It's important to remember that keeping glucose levels within a healthy range is key in preventing or delaying complications associated with diabetes.

If you can't determine why your glucose levels are elevated, or they continue to rise, contact your physician right away to understand the best treatment strategy in order to prevent levels from becoming dangerously high, which may lead to a condition known as *diabetic ketoacidosis.* In this condition, glucose levels rise due to the absence of insulin in the body. Although large amounts of glucose are in the bloodstream, glucose is unable to enter the cells for energy. Your cells, starved for energy, turn toward stored fat to break down for an energy alternative. Breaking down fat for energy results in the production of ketones as a waste product of this process. As ketones build in the body, they can throw off the body's acid/base balance, which can have serious health repercussions. If left untreated, this condition can lead to seizures, coma, and even death.

When glucose levels are elevated, such as after consuming a meal with a large amount of carbohydrates, one of the best ways to bring your levels back to a healthy range more quickly is to exercise. Simply walking after a meal can have a large impact on preventing or correcting hyperglycemia.

However, because ketoacidosis is a real risk, especially for individuals with type 1 diabetes, there are times that exercising with elevated glucose levels is not appropriate. Speak to your healthcare team about the appropriate recommendations for you. Many times a glucose level above 250mg/dL (milligrams of glucose per deciliter of blood) or 300mg/dL will require you to postpone exercise until your levels come back down into a healthy range.

## Taking hypoglycemia precautions

Because exercise can help to lower glucose levels in your bloodstream by using an increased amount of glucose for energy in the muscle cells as well as making your cells more sensitive to insulin, it's possible that your glucose levels may become _too_ low, a condition called _hypoglycemia._ Hypoglycemia is classified as a glucose level under 70mg/dL.

When glucose drops below this level, the condition must be treated to prevent it from continuing to drop, which can lead to serious health consequences such as seizures, unconsciousness, or even death.

If you are controlling type 2 diabetes through diet and exercise alone and are not on any form of medication, the chances of your glucose levels falling to dangerously low levels are rare. However, if you're on medication to lower glucose levels, especially insulin, you need to familiarize yourself with the signs and symptoms of hypoglycemia and know how to treat it before getting started with your exercise routine. If you catch the symptoms of hypoglycemia and treat it early, you can help prevent dangerous health consequences.

To prevent and treat hypoglycemia, make sure to check your blood glucose levels before and after exercise (as well as during exercise if you plan to walk for one hour or longer at one time). Although exercise can have an immediate effect on dropping test glucose levels, it can continue to drop them for as much as 18 hours after you stop exercising. Therefore, frequent monitoring when you first start exercising, or change an exercise routine, is very important so that you can understand how your body responds to exercise.

To prevent a dangerous drop in glucose levels, if your glucose levels are less than 100mg/dL before starting to exercise, have a carbohydrate-based snack (about 15 to 30 grams of carbohydrate) before getting started to protect yourself against a low.

At the completion of your walk, check your glucose levels and continue to do so every few hours after exercise. In addition, if you experience any symptoms of hypoglycemia, check your glucose right away. Some signs and symptoms include the following:

✔ Shakiness

✔ Cold sweat

✔ Fatigue

✔ General weakness

✔ Confusion

✔ Lack of coordination

✔ Slurred speech

✔ Irritability or anxiousness

If you feel as though you are beginning to experience any of these symptoms, stop exercising and check your glucose levels. If they have fallen below 70mg/dL, implement the *15-15 Rule* to correct hypoglycemia:

1. **Consume 15 grams of a fast-acting carbohydrate.**

   Four ounces of juice, four glucose tablets, or 8 ounces of soda is a good choice.

2. **Wait 15 minutes and retest your glucose levels.**

   If they are still below 70mg/dL, repeat this process until they are within a healthy range.

3. **Once glucose levels are in a healthy range, plan a meal or snack within one hour.**

   If the next meal or snack will be farther off, consume a snack containing about 15 grams of carbohydrate and 1 ounce of protein, such as 1 ounce of lowfat cheese on five whole-grain crackers, to prevent glucose from dropping yet again.

If you are at risk for hypoglycemia, you should always carry a fast-acting carbohydrate with you and wear a medical identification bracelet, identifying yourself as someone with diabetes.

# Walking with Prediabetes

Prediabetes is essentially a precursor to type 2 diabetes. You may have heard the terms *insulin resistant* or *impaired glucose tolerance,* which mean the same thing: Your body is becoming resistant to insulin. Glucose is starting to rise in the bloodstream, and if left untreated, most likely will result in a diagnosis of type 2 diabetes. Prediabetes affects a large number of adults (and even children and teens) in America. And although this condition can increase your risk for other conditions such as heart disease, you can think of it as an early warning as well. When you find out that you have prediabetes, your body is giving you a heads up that if you don't start making changes to your lifestyle now, you may just end up diagnosed with diabetes.

The good news is that through small, simple lifestyle changes, you can decrease insulin resistance, lower glucose levels, and avoid or delay a diagnosis of type 2 diabetes. But you have to take action and put in the work to make that happen.

## The impact of walking on insulin resistance

You can think of insulin as the key that opens up the cells and allows glucose in. With insulin resistance, the key doesn't fit into the lock. This predicament forces insulin, and with it, glucose, to remain in the bloodstream where they elevate over time. However, exercise is like a locksmith. With increased physical activity, the insulin "key" fits in the cells once again and can reopen them, allowing glucose back in and removing it from the bloodstream.

The more you walk and the more often you walk, the more your cells become sensitive to insulin again. Even just a few minutes per day can make a big difference when it comes to decreasing insulin resistance and preventing elevated glucose levels.

## Walking to prevent type 2 diabetes

Because insulin resistance is the main cause of type 2 diabetes, partaking in a behavior that reduces and reverses insulin resistance can help to prevent or delay a diagnosis of type 2 diabetes. Physical activity is one behavior that can make one of the largest impacts on preventing and correcting insulin resistance. First, being physically active can make the cells in your body more sensitive to insulin, helping it to reenter your cells. In addition, physical activity can help you achieve and maintain a healthy body weight, which also fights against insulin resistance.

One additional way being physically active helps is by reducing stress levels. The more stress you experience, the more your body produces counter-regulatory hormones that can elevate glucose levels. Exercise, however, can help to reduce stress in the body by releasing *endorphins,* or feel-good chemicals, in the brain, which help you to feel calm and relaxed and help to reduce circulating stress hormones in the body. Reducing stress levels can also fight against an accumulation of belly fat, which can increase the risk of a diagnosis of diabetes.

Take a look at the Diabetes Prevention Program study (`https://dppos.bsc.gwu.edu/`) to see just how little walking is needed to make a huge difference in the prevention of type 2 diabetes. In this study, individuals who had already been diagnosed with prediabetes worked to reduce body weight and increase physical activity through walking. By walking as little as 30 minutes per day and losing just 5–7 percent of their body weight (which is only 10 pounds for someone weighing 200 pounds), the participants were found to reduce their risk of developing diabetes by as much as 58 percent. As you can see, those small changes really do make a big difference when it comes to improving health.

# Walking and Weight Management with Diabetes

Achieving and maintaining a healthy body weight is key to helping maintain healthy glucose levels. With diabetes, the goal is to keep your glucose levels in a healthy range to prevent or delay complications associated with the disease. By working toward a healthy body weight, and maintaining that weight, you make it easier on yourself to keep your glucose within an ideal range and thus lower your odds of developing complications associated with the disease.

If you have weight to lose, becoming more physically active is one of the best ways to shed pounds and keep them off. The more you move, the more calories you burn. Because it takes 3,500 calories to burn off 1 pound of body fat, walking enough to burn 100 extra calories per day (about 1 mile per day above your normal day-to-day activity) can result in you losing almost 1 extra pound per month, or over 10 pounds in a year. Given that losing as little as 5 percent of your total body weight can make your body less resistant to insulin and provide better glucose outcomes, you can see just how quickly walking can make an impact on your waistline and your glucose management.

It's important to note that people with diabetes are also at an increased risk for other health conditions. For instance, those diagnosed with diabetes are four times more likely to suffer a heart attack or stroke. Being physically active, however, not only can help improve the management of diabetes, but can also help to prevent health risks such as heart disease as well. If you have diabetes, you can't afford not to start walking. But just make sure you do so safely. Always consult your physician before starting or changing any exercise routine. Also, make sure to monitor your glucose frequently before, during, and after exercise. Always carry a quick-acting carbohydrate with you in case of low glucose levels, and wear a medical ID bracelet identifying yourself as a person with diabetes. Walking can have many positive outcomes on diabetes as long as you take the necessary precautions to walk safely.

# Precautions for Those with Diabetes

In addition to taking precautions necessary to avoid or treat hypoglycemia when walking (see the earlier section "Taking hypoglycemia precautions"), it's also important that you take note of a few additional precautions you may not have considered before you get started. Diabetes can decrease circulation in the body, specifically to the lower extremities, such as your feet and toes. Decreased circulation can slow wound healing, so taking care to prevent and treat any injuries is vital in preventing infection.

Elevated glucose levels over time can cause a variety of complications such as heart disease, decline in kidney function, nerve damage *(neuropathy),* and damage to the retina of the eye *(retinopathy).* If you have been diagnosed with any of these conditions, you may need to take extra precautions as you get started with a walking routine. Speak with your physician about what forms of exercise, and the intensity of exercise, that may or may not be appropriate for you. If you have heart disease, make sure to read Chapter 13 for guidelines on how to walk safely with this condition to improve your heart health and prevent any negative consequences.

## Neuropathy and walking

Neuropathy occurs when nerves within your body are damaged, rendering them incapable of performing their normal functions. There are four main types of neuropathy you may experience from elevated glucose levels over time:

- ✔ **Peripheral neuropathy:** Nerve damage to extremities such as the toes, feet, hands, and arms

- ✔ **Autonomic neuropathy:** Damage to the nerves that regulate bowel, bladder, and digestive functions as well as heart and sexual functions

- ✔ **Proximal neuropathy:** Nerve damage to large nerves in the buttocks, hips, and thighs

- ✔ **Focal neuropathy:** Sudden weakness of a group of nerves; may occur anywhere within the body

Peripheral neuropathy poses the largest concern when it comes to exercising safely. This form of neuropathy can cause muscle weakness and a decrease in reflexes that may change your balance, gait, or even mobility. Because this can impact your steadiness on your feet, you may be at a higher risk for falls with this condition. For that reason, making sure to walk on a level surface is critical to creating a safe walking environment for yourself.

Neuropathy can lead to numbness in areas of the body, such as on the bottoms of the feet, so good foot care is vital in preventing wounds, which may be slow to heal or may become infected. For these reasons, before walking, make sure that you have properly fitting footwear to prevent irritation and blisters to your feet. Make sure you never walk barefooted and always inspect your shoes before putting them on to make sure there's no debris inside, such as a small stone, that could irritate your foot or cause injury. Inspect your feet every day looking for areas of redness, irritation, open wounds, or inflammation. If you discover an open wound or irritation, consult your physician right away for proper treatment to prevent infection. Because diabetes can lead to slow wound healing, an infection can become severe and, in extreme cases, can result in amputation. So be vigilant about your foot care so that you can continue to walk safely.

## Retinopathy and walking

Retinopathy is a disease that affects the retina of the eye, which results in impairment or loss of vision. This condition is the number-one cause of new blindness in adults in America and a major risk factor for anyone with diabetes, especially those who struggle to maintain healthy glucose levels. With this condition, blood vessels in the eye can swell, leak, and even bleed. However, the good news is that research has not found aerobic exercise to worsen this condition. Nevertheless, with diabetes, you should see your ophthalmologist annually for a full vision screening and if any changes in vision occur, you should see your eye doctor more often.

If blood pressure is elevated, it can make retinopathy more severe. Therefore, exercises that cause you to strain, such as heavy weight lifting, should be avoided to prevent a rise in blood pressure, which may cause further damage to the eye. Because of this, speak to your physician before starting any of the exercise plans in this book — especially before incorporating any of the strength-training exercises — to make sure they are appropriate for you and safe to perform based on your individual condition. High-intensity exercise as well as any exercise that increases the risk of injury to the eye, such as contact sports or kickboxing, should also be avoided.

# Maximizing Your Walking Workout with Diabetes

Just because you have been diagnosed with diabetes doesn't mean that you can't increase the intensity of your walking workout over time. However, you must be careful to do so safely. The longer and more intensely you exercise, the greater your risk of experiencing hypoglycemia, or low glucose levels. In addition, if you have complications from diabetes, such as neuropathy, retinopathy, or heart disease, extra care needs to be taken when planning your walking routine to avoid any risk of injury or medical complications.

Before adding incline, interval training, or resistance to your walking workout, make sure to speak to your physician about what forms of exercise and intensity are most appropriate for you. Then, make sure to follow these guidelines for a safe and enjoyable walking workout:

✓ Walk on even surfaces to prevent the risk of falls.

✓ Wear properly fitted footwear that provides the appropriate amount of support.

✓ Inspect your feet daily and contact your healthcare provider at the first signs of foot irritation, wounds, or infection.

✓ Check your glucose levels before, during, and after exercise to prevent hypoglycemia.

✓ Familiarize yourself with the signs and symptoms of hypoglycemia and make sure to check your glucose levels at the first sign of symptoms.

✓ Speak to your healthcare team about your individual glucose targets and what glucose ranges may be too low or too high to safely exercise at.

✓ Always carry a fast-acting carbohydrate with you to treat hypoglycemia if needed.

✓ Wear a medical ID bracelet.

# Chapter 13

# Walking Away Heart Disease

* * * * * * * * * * * * * * * * * * * * * * * * * * * * * * * * * * * * * *

* * * * * * * * * * * * * * * * * * * * * * * * * * * * * * * * * * * * * *

Heart disease is the number one killer among both men and women in America. In fact, 49 percent of all American adults have at least one major risk factor for heart disease. If you have elevated cholesterol levels, high blood pressure, or elevated blood glucose levels, you are at an increased risk for heart disease. If you're a smoker, overweight, or lead an inactive lifestyle, you are also at an increased risk for heart disease. Your heart is a muscle, and just like any muscle, if you want to keep it strong, you need to exercise it.

Regular walking can help to reduce almost all the most common risk factors for heart disease. By following the walking plans in this book, you can lose weight and shed inches off your waistline, helping to reduce your odds of heart disease. In addition, regular movement helps to lower blood pressure, blood glucose, and cholesterol levels, all helping to further protect your heart.

In fact, walking just 30 minutes per day has been shown to lower the risk of developing heart disease by as much as 30 to 40 percent! Instead of becoming another statistic, just put one foot in front of the other and get moving. The more you walk, the stronger and healthier your heart will become.

# The Link Between Inactivity and Heart Disease

Being inactive can lead to a cascade of unhealthy events in your body. Inactivity can lead to increased body weight and increased storage of dangerous belly fat, or visceral fat. Even if you are at a healthy body weight, if your waistline slowly expands over time from inactivity, your risk for heart disease increases. A 4-inch increase in waist circumference has been associated with a 15 percent higher chance of developing heart disease — even if you are already at a healthy body weight.

Even if your waistline doesn't expand, the link between inactivity and an increased risk for heart disease is strong. Study after study shows that regular movement is essential in keeping all of your vital organs healthy and preventing disease. In fact, you can't afford not to walk when it comes to your health and well-being. Walking can help to improve your cardiovascular fitness, improve the flexibility of your arteries, and even help to lower stress hormones that can negatively impact the function of your heart.

## Understanding the need to take care of your heart

Your heart is one of the most vital organs, if not the most vital organ, in your entire body. It's a powerful muscle that is constantly pumping blood, oxygen, and essential nutrients to all the cells of your body. If your heart ceases to function, life can only be sustained for a few minutes. A poorly functioning heart impacts all the organs of your body as circulation decreases, oxygen and blood take longer to reach your cells, and blood vessels stiffen. In order to not only increase longevity but also quality of life, keeping your heart functioning at its peak is essential.

Coronary artery disease occurs as plaque builds up in the arteries, causing them to stiffen. This buildup in turn makes it more difficult for blood to travel through the blood vessels, forcing your heart to work harder and harder. The harder your heart has to work to pump blood through the body, the higher your blood pressure goes and the weaker your heart becomes over time. However, by just increasing your overall movement day after day, you can fight against plaque buildup and allow blood to flow quickly and easily throughout your body. In fact, research has found that when individuals in their 50s and 60s walked just 45 to 60 minutes per day, their hearts were more effective at pumping blood and nutrients. In fact, their hearts were so much more effective, they were functioning on the level of individuals in their

30s! You really can turn back the clock when it comes to your health and your heart, but it all starts with getting more active. And the easiest and most effective way to do that is — you guessed it — by walking!

## Determining whether walking is right for you

As you can see, moving more is key when it comes to the fight against heart disease. Although any form of exercise can help to improve heart health, walking is thought to be the perfect exercise in managing and preventing heart disease for a variety of reasons. For one, walking is a low-intensity exercise, which means you can determine just how hard you want to push yourself. If you already have heart disease, you may have some exercise restrictions, such as keeping your heart rate within a target range. Because higher-intensity exercises, such as jogging, often elevate heart rate quickly, you may find sticking to your target range more challenging with such an exercise. Instead, with walking, you can walk at a slow, leisurely rate and keep your heart rate in check while still gaining the benefits of daily exercise.

Being consistent with exercise is vital in fighting against heart disease. If you only exercise once or twice per week, you may not see much improvement in the risk factors for heart disease, such as blood pressure or cholesterol levels. High-intensity exercises can lead to injury or even burnout, making it harder to be consistent. Instead, walking is something you can do anywhere, at any time, with any level of intensity you choose. For this reason, it's much easier to be consistent and stick with your walking routine.

Walking is also a perfect activity for preventing heart disease as it takes little skill, mostly because you already do it every day. An exercise that is simple to do is an exercise you can get started with right away. Say you decide to take up dancing to increase your physical fitness. That's a terrific exercise and a great way to improve cardiovascular health. However, you first need to find a space to dance, learn various dance steps, perhaps work with a dance instructor, and so on. By the time you get started and feel comfortable with the exercise itself, days or even weeks may have passed. Instead, with walking, you can get started right now. All you have to do is place one foot in front of the other, and you can start walking for exercise anyplace, anytime.

# How Walking Can Benefit Your Heart

In order to gain control of your heart health, first you have to understand your risk factors for heart disease. Although this disease is incredibly widespread, there are multiple factors that can increase your individual risk.

Once you identify your own personal risk factors for heart disease, you can start taking the steps needed to decrease your overall risk. Key risk factors for heart disease include the following:

- ✔ Elevated blood pressure levels
- ✔ Elevated LDL cholesterol
- ✔ Low HDL cholesterol
- ✔ Elevated triglycerides
- ✔ Elevated blood glucose levels
- ✔ Elevated C-reactive protein
- ✔ Elevated homocysteine levels
- ✔ Overweight or obese
- ✔ Wide waistline
- ✔ Smoker
- ✔ Sedentary lifestyle

If you look closely at the list of risk factors for heart disease, almost every single one can be prevented, managed, and even reversed with physical activity. For instance, British researchers found that by just walking for 30 minutes five days a week, C-reactive protein levels could be significantly reduced. And at times, walking may help to reverse the risk factors for heart disease even more so than other forms of exercise. For instance, one study found that walkers were able to lower their levels of triglycerides almost twice as much as joggers who exercised for the same amount of time and with the same frequency.

The longer you walk, the more often you walk, and the more you stay consistent with your walking workout, the more you'll reap the benefits of walking when it comes to heart health.

## Walking and blood pressure

One of the largest risk factors for heart disease is having an elevated blood pressure, also known as *hypertension,* which is a condition that impacts about 78 million Americans. Blood pressure is essentially the measurement of the pressure the blood exerts on your vessels as it's pumped throughout the body. The higher your blood pressure, the harder your heart must work to pump blood, oxygen, and nutrients throughout the day, weakening it over time. Having an elevated blood pressure level dramatically increases the risk for heart attack and stroke. The goal for blood pressure is to keep it at 120/80 millimeters of mercury or below. Hypertension, or elevated blood pressure, is defined by the American Heart Association as having a *systolic* (or upper number) blood pressure at or above 140 millimeters of mercury or a *diastolic* (or lower number) blood pressure at or above 90 millimeters of mercury.

When working to reduce blood pressure, diet can play a key role. Diets rich in saturated fats, sodium, and refined carbohydrates can trigger an increase in blood pressure levels. On the other hand, a low-sodium diet rich in fresh fruit, vegetables, and whole grains can help to reduce blood pressure. But it's not just diet that plays a role in blood pressure management. Exercise, such as walking, is critical in bringing this number down. In fact, researchers have spent decade after decade trying to develop new treatments to reduce blood pressure levels, and yet exercise is still shown to be one of the very best ways to manage this condition.

Exercise is so powerful in the fight against hypertension that just one work-out can help to reduce blood pressure levels for an entire day. And exercising on a regular basis can reduce blood pressure and keep it under control long term. And it doesn't take much to make an impact! Individuals with hypertension who had previously been sedentary were able to significantly reduce their blood pressure levels with just small amounts of physical activity. Just 60 to 90 minutes of exercise during the week was enough to make a big impact on blood pressure levels. If you average that over the course of a week, that's less than 10 minutes per day of walking. By just adding that small amount of extra activity to your day, you can start to see positive changes in your blood pressure levels.

When it comes to lowering blood pressure, the more you can walk, the better. In the American Heart Association's journal *Hypertension,* researchers found walking four hours or more per week was found to lower blood pressure by as much as 20 percent. But even doing just one to three hours of leisure exercise per week brought blood pressure 11 percent lower than engaging in less than one hour of activity per week. Research has also found that low- to moderate-intensity exercise, such as walking, may be even more beneficial to reducing blood pressure levels than higher-intensity exercise. As you can see, if you have or are at risk of having elevated blood pressure levels, walking, even just for a few minutes per day, can make a significant impact on your overall heart health.

## Walking and blood lipids

Blood lipids are made up of your total cholesterol, which includes LDL cholesterol (or "lousy" cholesterol), HDL cholesterol (or "happy" cholesterol), and triglycerides. A favorable blood lipid panel for heart disease prevention includes reduced total cholesterol, LDL cholesterol, and triglyceride levels with an elevated HDL cholesterol. Having unfavorable cholesterol levels can make you two times more likely to develop heart disease. About 71 million Americans have elevated LDL cholesterol levels, yet only one in three have this condition under control.

Although diet can play a large role in your blood lipid panel, exercise can make a huge impact as well. Just by walking small amounts each day, you can see a dramatic improvement in total cholesterol and LDL cholesterol reduction, while helping to increase HDL cholesterol levels. Research has found that walking just 12 miles per week can significantly improve blood lipids by helping to reduce LDL cholesterol levels as well as total cholesterol levels. When you increase the amount of exercise further, such as by walking 20 miles per week (which averages out to just under 3 miles per day), HDL cholesterol can also be significantly increased, providing further protection to your heart. Just by being physically active and walking more, you can decrease your risk for coronary artery disease by as much as 45 percent.

# Planning Your Walking Routine with Heart Disease

If you have been diagnosed with heart disease, you may be wondering whether walking is appropriate for you. You may be concerned about becoming physically active and how increasing your movement, and therefore your heart rate, may impact your overall heart health. Although regular exercise can decrease the risk of developing heart disease, if you've already been diagnosed with this disease, you need to take some additional precautions before getting started with an exercise plan.

Before starting or changing any exercise routine, especially if you have been diagnosed with heart disease or are at an increased risk for developing it, you should see your doctor. Your doctor can evaluate your current health situation and let you know what forms of exercise are and are not safe for you at this time. He can also inform you of any heart-rate-range goals you may need to monitor or any additional guidelines you need to follow.

Even with heart disease, getting active is still important and recommended. If you have heart disease, being inactive puts you at a greater risk of worsening the disease. Being inactive can also negatively impact many of the factors that contribute to worsening heart disease, such as blood pressure, cholesterol, diabetes, and being overweight. However, as little as 30 minutes of low- to moderate-intensity exercise, such as walking, most days of the week can protect your heart and make it stronger, younger, and healthier. In fact, just this small amount of exercise lessens your likelihood of having a stroke, developing diabetes, having elevated blood pressure levels, or suffering a heart attack.

When it comes to walking away heart disease, you can gain health benefits even if you can't perform 30 minutes of exercise all at once. Cumulative exercise is beneficial when it comes to improving your overall heart health. If walking for 30 minutes at once seems taxing on your body, break it up. Taking three ten-minute walks throughout the day may be much more manageable while providing you with all the same health benefits.

## Taking precautions with heart disease

In addition to consulting your physician before starting or changing a walking workout, there are a few other precautions to consider before you begin your exercise routine if you have been diagnosed with heart disease. Taking these precautions into consideration will help to protect you from any negative implications of exercise, so you can focus instead on all the benefits walking will bring to your body, your weight, and your overall health.

When it comes to safely exercising, consider any changes that may occur that can impact your walking workout. For instance, if you have started a new medication or your medications have recently been changed, make sure to call your doctor to discuss how this change in medication may impact your planned exercise routine. Don't start or continue with your workout plan until you've discussed any changes or additions in medications with your physician.

With heart disease, it's important to continue to assess how you are feeling before, during, and after exercise. For instance, if you're feeling overly tired or weak some days, look at what you did the day before. Did you try and push yourself to exercise too long or too hard? If so, you may need to scale back and increase the intensity of your exercise routine gradually to prevent overexertion. As you walk, watch your breathing. If you become short of breath, stop walking and relax for a short period of time by standing still or sitting comfortably until you can catch your breath again. Do the same if you become overly fatigued while walking. Pushing through is not helpful and may be dangerous. Instead, allow yourself rest periods to make sure you're not straining too much.

When you are exercising, never ignore pain. If you develop chest pain or have pain in any part of your body, stop exercising and rest. Contact your physician or physical therapist for instructions on what may or may not be appropriate exercise for your body. You should also stop walking and rest if you develop any of the following symptoms at any time during your workout:

- Chest pain
- General weakness
- Dizziness or lightheadedness
- Pressure or pain in your chest, neck, arm, jaw, or shoulder

If these symptoms continue, consult your physician right away.

## Recognizing restrictions with heart disease

Walking is a great way to strengthen your heart and to prevent complications associated with heart disease. However, with this condition, there are a few restrictions to note when it comes to increasing your activity level. By understanding these restrictions, you can ensure you are exercising safely and not increasing your risk for complications.

As you get started with your walking workout, take note of the temperature before doing your workout outdoors. If it's too cold, too hot, or too humid, it may be best to avoid exercising outside as this can impact circulation, making breathing more difficult and possibly causing chest pain. Instead, on days such as this, do your workout indoors in a temperature-regulated space, such as walking on a treadmill or mall walking. And just as extreme temperatures are not preferable during a walk, they should be avoided after your workout as well. Try to avoid very hot or very cold showers, baths, or even saunas and hot tubs after your workout as well.

Although you may want to push yourself to burn more calories and intensify your workout, if you have heart disease, you need to be careful in your approach to doing so. Consider the following:

- Lifting or pushing heavy objects, such as lifting heavy dumbbells, should be avoided.
- Avoid performing push-ups, sit-ups, and isometric exercises to prevent straining that can increase heart rate and blood pressure levels.
- If you want to add resistance to your walking workout, do so by using only lightweight objects, such as resistance bands, and get your physician's clearance before starting.

✔ Adding incline, such as walking up a steep hill, is also contraindicated with heart disease, as this may raise your heart rate too high. Instead, walk on a flat surface and, if you need to increase your workout's intensity, try walking for a longer duration or slightly increasing your walking speed.

Keep a close eye on your heart rate any time you increase your workout intensity and follow your physician's guidelines as to what range your heart rate should stay within.

If you have had to stop exercising for three or more days, don't jump back in right where you left off. Instead, scale down the intensity of your walk (by walking for a shorter distance, less time, or at a lower speed) and gradually increase back up to your regular exercise level over a few days to avoid stressing your heart. As you exercise, make sure to slow down or rest if you become short of breath or experience fatigue at any time. As you rest, elevate your feet and if your shortness of breath continues, contact your physician. If at any point you develop a rapid or irregular heart beat or feel heart palpitations, rest, relax, and check your pulse. If your pulse stays above 120 to 150 beats per minute after 15 minutes of rest, call your physician.

# Maximizing Your Workout with Heart Disease

In Chapter 11, I outline ways that you can maximize your walking workout to burn more calories and body fat. However, some ways to intensify your workout are not always appropriate if you have been diagnosed with heart disease.

Adding an incline or adding a large amount of resistance may cause a dangerous spike in your heart rate and should be avoided if you have heart disease. But this doesn't mean that you can't challenge yourself with your walking workout for faster results. You just have to make sure the way in which you do it is appropriate for you and your heart condition.

First, before changing your walking workout, speak to your doctor. Discuss what you would like to do during your workout and whether it's appropriate for you. Ask whether you have any exercise restrictions and whether you should be monitoring your heart rate during exercise. If heart rate monitoring is recommended, ask your physician what range she would prefer that you keep your heart rate within.

Although adding an incline or resistance exercising to your walking workout may be contraindicated for your specific health needs, you can still increase the amount of calories you burn during your walking workout. One of the easiest ways to do this is by increasing the duration of your walk. You can keep your walking speed consistent, but just walk a few additional minutes each day. This strategy allows you to walk a greater distance and, therefore, burn more calories and fat.

If you've been given heart rate guidelines for your walking workout, make sure to wear a heart rate monitor throughout the duration of your workout. As you wear your monitor, you can continue to verify that what you're doing for exercise is not bringing you outside of your target heart rate range. As you walk, you can start to increase your speed over time. If, for instance, you walk a mile in 25 minutes, aim to walk the same mile in 24 minutes, and then when that becomes easy enough, increase your speed to do it in 23 minutes. As long as you can increase your speed gradually over time without spiking your heart rate out of its ideal range, you can safely increase the intensity of your walk.

You can also use this same technique to add interval training to your walk. With interval training, you walk at a slower speed for a set length of time — for instance, five minutes — followed by walking at a faster speed for a short time, such as 30 seconds, and repeating. You can practice this technique as long as you monitor your heart rate throughout the exercise. When you incorporate interval training, make sure to introduce it gradually. The shorter, faster walking periods should only be fast enough to challenge yourself without raising your heart rate outside of your ideal zone.

With careful monitoring and clearance from your physician, and by taking a gradual approach to adjusting your workout, you can increase the intensity and maximize your results while keeping your heart safe and healthy.

# Chapter 14

# Walking Your Belly and Butt Off

If you've picked up this book, you're most likely looking to lose weight. And if you're like most people, you want to shed inches from your thighs, backside, and midsection. These areas of your body tend to cling to fat stores, making it challenging to tone and tighten these areas. However, slimming your waistline, your buttocks, and your thighs can make a marked difference in the way your clothes fit, the way you feel, and most importantly, your health.

Although visceral fat, or belly fat, as it's commonly called, is something most of us look to shed for vanity reasons, getting rid of this stubborn fat is also essential for good health.

Excess belly fat is one of the most dangerous forms of fat, because this fat isn't just stored energy. It's metabolically active, meaning that it constantly produces hormones and chemicals in your body. The close proximity of belly fat to vital organs causes these organs to become overexposed to these chemicals and hormones, damaging them and increasing your risk for a multitude of health conditions such as heart disease, diabetes, and even certain cancers. Walking, however, can help you shed this dangerous fat so you not only look and feel better, but are healthier as well.

## Walking to Reduce Belly Fat

In addition to your food choices, exercise plays a very large role in helping reduce belly fat, but not only for the reasons you may think. Exercise, as I am sure you know, burns calories, which in turn can help promote weight loss. But that's not the only way exercise impacts belly fat. Exercise plays a large role in stress reduction by reducing the stress response and releasing endorphins in the brain, which help improve mood and decrease overall stress levels. Physical activity also helps reduce insulin resistance. When insulin resistance is reduced, your body is better able to handle sugar, and your pancreas may need to produce less insulin to keep blood sugar levels in check. Since you now know how excess insulin in the bloodstream can promote increased belly fat storage, you can see why this is helpful.

Need one last reason to get moving? Exercise can boost your metabolism — and not just when you are exercising! When you strengthen and build muscle during exercise, especially during resistance exercise, you rev up your metabolism all day long, even when you're sleeping.

## Maintaining a consistent (and easy) routine

Becoming physically active can help your body to start shedding unwanted belly fat in a variety of ways. However, in order to gain the benefits of a slimmer waistline, you need to be consistent with your exercise routine. Although many forms of exercise can help you burn belly fat, walking is the only form of exercise that you can do pretty much anywhere, anytime, regardless of your age or experience level. For these reasons, walking is the most preferred form of exercise among individuals who have lost weight and kept it off long term.

Ask yourself this: If you were to start exercising today with a goal to exercise most days of the week, what would be the easiest, most convenient, and most affordable exercise to do? Can you think of any exercise that would be simpler, more accessible, and cheaper than walking? Walking really is the easiest exercise you can do. In addition, it's so versatile: You can walk briskly or slowly, uphill or on a flat surface, with resistance or without, and the list goes on. Because it's such a convenient exercise, it's easy to stick with, which is why it's one of the best ways to shed belly fat.

And walking isn't just easy to do. Research shows that it's incredibly effective at targeting the fat that you want to get rid of the most — belly fat! For example, a Canadian study found that simply walking for one hour a day led to a 20 percent reduction in belly fat in just 14 weeks! If walking for an hour a day seems like too much, think about this: Walking just 1 to 2 miles three times per week was shown in another study to shrink belly fat cells by as much as 18 percent over a four-month period! So not only does walking help you to shed pounds, it also targets the area of your body you are most concerned about. And it does so quickly, without a huge time commitment, helping you to stay motivated as well!

# Maximizing your walking workout

When it comes to targeting belly fat and shedding it for good, the combination of aerobic exercise with resistance training has been found to be the most effective at burning up this stubborn fat. That's where the walking plans such as the total body walking workout, the resistance walking workout, and the weight-loss maximizer workout (see Chapter 10 for more on these specific workouts) incorporate a combination of cardiovascular exercise in the form of brisk walking along with exercises to strengthen and tone all the major muscle groups in your body. The more muscle mass you build, the higher your metabolism goes, making shedding pounds and inches easier and keeping them off much more likely.

As you go through this book and browse through the various walking plans and programs, you'll see I often discuss interval training. Interval training pairs lower-intensity exercise with higher-intensity exercise, and that pattern is repeated throughout the duration of the workout. This form of exercise is the most effective way to target stubborn areas of fat, such as belly fat, and see faster results. Even if you're new to walking, you can incorporate small forms of interval training by walking slightly faster every five minutes during your walk, or adding a slight incline every ten minutes for 30 seconds or one minute. Even though these minor adjustments seem like small changes, they lead to huge results when it comes to shrinking your waistline.

# Keeping belly fat from returning

Shedding pounds and inches is just half the battle. The real fight comes in keeping that unwanted belly fat from returning. In order to lose weight and keep it off, you have to make lifestyle changes, not just changes you will stick with for a short period of time only to go back to old habits. That's why selecting an exercise like walking that can be done anywhere, anytime, with limited wear and tear on your body is so important. It's no wonder that 78 percent of individuals in the National Weight Control Registry, a registry of individuals who have lost at least 30 pounds and kept it off for more than a year, report walking as their preferred source of exercise.

Consistency is key when it comes to weight management. Consistently making healthy food choices and staying physically active are the ingredients you need to achieve and maintain a healthy body weight. With walking, it's easy to be consistent. First, you can break walking up throughout the day. For instance, walking for 10 minutes three times per day provides you with the same health and weight-loss benefits as walking for 30 minutes all at once. And it's easier to find a few 10-minute slots throughout the day than one large chunk of time to exercise.

In addition, walking isn't that taxing on your body. Because it's a low-impact exercise, there's less chance that you'll become sidelined with an injury, allowing you to keep up with walking on a regular basis. Plus, it's so versatile. You can change how you walk, where you walk, and even the speed and incline of your walk over and over again, keeping you from ever getting bored while challenging your body more and more.

# Walking Your Butt Off

Do you want to tone and tighten your backside? If your behind isn't what you hope for, you don't just have to live with it. You can actually tone and tighten your glutes to give your behind a firm and lifted appearance. And you can do it all simply by walking!

To tone your buttocks, you need to understand the muscles that make it up. Three gluteal muscles make up the buttocks area: the gluteus maximus, the gluteus medius, and the gluteus minimus. The gluteus maximus is the largest of these three muscles (thus its name), and it's positioned underneath the cheeks of your buttocks. The gluteus medius and minimus are located around the upper part of your hip bone. Together, these muscles work to provide stabilization to your entire body as well as to help extend your legs.

Because the gluteus maximus is the bulkiest skeletal muscle in your entire body, toning this muscle helps to define the shape of your bottom. In addition, strengthening this muscle has benefits beyond just physical appearance. A strong gluteus maximus increases the strength of your entire lower body and increases stability in your body as well. Every step you take when walking utilizes and tones this muscle group. However, if you really want to strengthen and define these muscles, specifically the gluteus maximus, a leisurely walk at a slow pace isn't going to help you make much headway. A brisk-paced walk, with fast, small steps, can help to boost strength, tone, and definition, allowing you to achieve the results you are aiming for.

## Tailoring your workout to target your glutes

When it comes to strengthening, toning, and shaping your bottom, brisk walking is key. When you walk quickly (a mile in under 15 minutes), you challenge all the gluteal muscles, helping them to become stronger and more defined. In addition, to maximize the results of a brisk walk, focus on tightening this muscle group as you walk. As you do this, take smaller steps to boost your speed and see results more quickly. In addition, adding an incline to your walk further strengthens and tones this area, providing you with even faster results. If you walk on a treadmill, raising the incline as little as 2 percent is enough to challenge this muscle group. A higher incline, such as walking up a steep hill or climbing stairs, further challenges these muscles and strengthens and tones them even more quickly.

Think about the walking plan you are currently following. Are you walking at a fast or slow pace? Are you walking on a flat surface or do you include an incline? Making just a few small adjustments to your current walk can help you to target your glutes and maximize your results. Try incorporating one, or all, of these strategies into your next walk to really get your glutes working:

- ✔ **Speed up your walk.** Time how long it takes you to walk one mile. Each time you walk, aim to complete one mile 30 seconds faster than the time before. Accelerate your pace by taking small, short, quick steps. Work toward a goal of finishing a mile in under 15 minutes for the most challenging workout for your glutes.

- ✔ **Head to the hills!** Adding an incline, even a very small one, automatically increases the burden on your gluteal muscles. Try adding a small hill to your typically outdoor walking route, increase the incline by 1 to 2 percent if you walk on a treadmill, or walk up and down the stairs while mall walking to gain these benefits.

- ✔ **Squeeze those glutes.** As you are walking, pay careful attention to your posture. Make sure to hold your upper body upright and keep your back straight and pull your abs in. While walking, tightly squeeze your gluteal muscles to challenge them to work harder. This strategy helps this muscle group to tone and tighten faster.

- ✔ **Add resistance.** Incorporate strength-training exercises that target the gluteal muscles during or after your walking workout. Lunges, leg raises, and glute bridges are all fantastic ways to challenge this muscle group for faster results. Check out the total body walking workout along with the resistance walking workout in Chapter 10 for exercises that target this area.

## *Toning your glutes while walking*

Adding speed, incline, or resistance are all effective ways to tone and tighten your gluteal muscles. You can add some or all of these forms of exercise to your walking routine to help you see results. But before you do, you want to decide which forms of exercise are best for you. If you're new to exercise and walking, you want to start out gradually to prevent excessive muscle soreness or injury. If you're a walking pro, you still want to take care to ensure you are gradually increasing the intensity of your workout to protect against burnout and injury.

If you choose to add incline to your walking workout, be cautious if you have any current or prior leg injuries, such as chronic knee pain or lower back pain. Walking at a steep incline may place more pressure on your back and knees, increasing pain and possibly increasing the risk of future injury. If this is the case, instead of adding an incline to your walking workout, focus on toning your gluteal muscles by tightening them during your workout, picking up your pace, and incorporating resistance exercises into your plan.

If you are new to exercise but looking to tone your glutes, get started gradually. Start by just timing your walk for a set distance, such as 1 mile or ½ mile. Whatever your time may be to complete the walk, work on increasing your speed to complete the same distance in 30 fewer seconds on the next walk, and continue to decrease the time it takes you to walk the same distance until you are walking at the rate of a 12–15 minute mile. You can also slowly start to add an incline to your workout. But again, add this gradually to protect yourself against injury. If you walk on a treadmill, add 1 percent incline and walk at this rate for one week. Then increase by 1 percent the next week and so on until you are walking at an incline you find challenging and can feel your glutes working.

If you don't have access to a treadmill, you can still increase your incline no matter where you walk. If you're outdoors, look to see whether you can change your walking route to one that offers a slight hill for a more challenging walk. You can also switch one or two of your weekly walking workouts to try an uphill hike to further challenge yourself. If you don't have access to hills, look for ways you can climb stairs during a walk, whether inside or outside. And even if you have no access to stairs, you can still challenge your gluteal muscles by adding lunges, either stationary or in motion, to your walk. The total body walking workout and the resistance walking workout show you how to incorporate lunges for a more toned and tightened backside.

# Chapter 15

# Walking During Pregnancy and Beyond

Congratulations on your pregnancy! Whether this is your first child or you are already a seasoned parent, pregnancy is an exciting but overwhelming time. You may be concerned about eating as healthily as possible or being as active as you can so that your unborn child will remain healthy and continue to thrive. In addition to the necessary planning that takes place leading up to your child's birth, trying to adjust your lifestyle to improve your health and that of your child's can at times seem overwhelming.

Staying or becoming physically active is an important part of a healthy pregnancy. Very high-intensity exercise and sports or exercises that have a risk of contact or fall are not recommended during this time, so finding a low- to moderate-intensity form of exercise you can perform throughout pregnancy — and again after childbirth — is a great way to keep up your energy level, boost your immune system, and have the healthiest pregnancy possible. Many moms have found themselves turning toward walking for exercise. This chapter takes a look at just why walking can be so great during pregnancy as well as shortly after.

# Staying Physically Active During Pregnancy

Whether you're already active or have been sedentary, getting and staying active during pregnancy can be incredibly beneficial to you as well as your unborn child. Regular walking throughout the duration of the pregnancy can help you stay healthy and feel your best. In fact, the more physically active you can be, the less fatigue you may experience during your pregnancy.

Many women, especially in the first trimester, find themselves feeling incredibly fatigued. If you are one of them, although it can be hard to talk yourself into exercise when you're feeling tired, getting active can give your energy levels and mood a lift.

In addition, physical activity on a regular basis can help fight off many of the most common discomforts during pregnancy. Because back pain is common, especially in the last trimester of pregnancy, an activity such as walking that helps to promote healthy posture can help. Staying active can also decrease your risks for developing complications such as gestational diabetes and hypertension (high blood pressure) during your pregnancy. And being active from your first trimester through the end of your third trimester can help you build the strength and stamina you need to get through labor and delivery. Stress levels can be elevated during pregnancy. The stress of getting prepared for the baby and setting up the nursery, the anxiety of the unknown when it comes to labor and delivery, the stress of picking out a baby name or figuring out how to manage your work schedule, childcare, and the list of to-dos that come with having a baby can all add up. This stress can be hard to manage; however, regular exercise can help.

Walking releases endorphins, those feel-good chemicals in the brain that elevate your mood and allow you to better handle stress. In addition, regular exercise lowers the stress hormones that your body secretes when you start to feel overwhelmed. High stress levels aren't healthy for you or your baby, so finding ways to relieve and manage stress, such as walking, is key to a healthy pregnancy.

## Determining whether walking is appropriate for you

Walking throughout and after your pregnancy can have many positive effects for both you and your baby. But you do first want to make sure that walking is appropriate for you. Before starting or changing any exercise routine, especially if you are already pregnant, make sure to discuss this issue with your physician or obstetrician.

If yours is considered a high-risk pregnancy, you may need to be monitored more closely or follow restrictions on the amount, type, or intensity of exercise you may perform. Always follow your doctor's instructions when it comes to exercise during and after pregnancy.

For most individuals, if you were already exercising before becoming pregnant, you may continue with your regular exercise routine as long as the activity is moderate in intensity and doesn't include contact sports or have a high chance of falling. For instance, sports like kickboxing or skiing aren't recommended during pregnancy due to the potential of harm to the baby if you were to fall or if direct contact were to be made with the baby. Most doctors recommend that you also keep an eye on your heart rate while exercising during pregnancy and avoid allowing it to elevate above 140 beats per minute. Scaling down the intensity of an exercise if your heart rate exceeds this amount is recommended to prevent an elevated body temperature, which can impact your baby.

If you have never exercised before, you can safely start to increase your physical activity level, but only after discussing it with your doctor first. If you are starting to exercise during pregnancy, this isn't the time to try out very strenuous or high-intensity exercise programs. Instead, you want to elevate your overall activity level and exercise at a low to moderate intensity. Walking allows you to do just that and is thought to be the safest form of exercise when starting to exercise during pregnancy.

## Deciding how much walking is safe during pregnancy

Just as no two babies are exactly alike, no two pregnancies or mothers are either. How often and how much you can and should walk during pregnancy depend on a variety of factors. Were you already walking or exercising regularly before becoming pregnant? Do you have any pregnancy complications or is your pregnancy considered high risk? Are you carrying multiple babies (twins, triplets, or more) or just one? Are you experiencing extreme fatigue, nausea, or other ill effects of pregnancy?

Depending on your activity level before pregnancy, how you feel during your pregnancy, and the health of your pregnancy, walking recommendations vary. The recommendation from the American College of Obstetrics and Gynecology is to perform moderate exercise, such as walking, for 30 minutes or more most, if not all, days of the week — unless, of course, you have any medical or obstetric complications or have been advised differently by your physician.

Because pregnancy is not the time to exhaust yourself or push yourself to your limits physically, starting gradually is important, especially if you are new to exercise. Aim to walk just a few minutes per day at first and see how you feel. You can add 5 minutes to your walk each day until you can comfortably walk 30 minutes at once. Or you can break your walk into three ten-minute walks per day if this is more manageable for you. Later in your pregnancy, you may find breaking your walks into smaller segments helpful if you experience any discomfort, such as back pain or swollen feet and ankles.

## Choosing the right intensity level for your walking routine

If you were already exercising before becoming pregnant, you can continue on with your exercise routine. However, high-intensity or high-impact exercise is often not recommended during pregnancy, to prevent excess stress on you and your baby. A lower-intensity form of exercise, such as walking, is safe to continue throughout your pregnancy.

Throughout your pregnancy, sometimes you have more or less energy than at other times. Sometimes you experience discomfort, and other times you feel great. Listen to your body when it comes to exercise and don't push yourself beyond what feels comfortable. If you feel short of breath, weak, dizzy, or have discomfort at any time while exercising, stop and rest. If these symptoms persist, contact your physician for further instructions.

Monitoring your heart rate while exercising during pregnancy can be a helpful way to ensure you are not exercising too intensely. The rule of thumb is to keep your heart rate below 140 beats per minute. If you exceed this, lower the intensity of the exercise slightly until you are safely in this range.

Pay attention to perceived exertion as well. Never exercise to the point where you are so out of breath that you can barely speak. Although it's safe to walk at a speed at which you can't speak in full sentences, you should always be able to speak a few words comfortably. If this isn't possible, lower the intensity of your exercise.

# Exercising Safely During Pregnancy

For most women, exercise is safe during pregnancy. In fact, most physicians encourage regular exercise due to the benefits it offers to both the mother and unborn child.

However, for pregnancies that are considered high risk for complications or for mothers with conditions such as elevated blood pressure, exercise may need to be limited or restricted.

Before jumping into an exercise routine or continuing with the exercise you were doing before pregnancy, have a discussion with your physician about what is most appropriate for you. When speaking to your doctor, outline what type of exercise, like walking, you want to do, how often you plan to do it, and the average intensity level of your workout. Then, ask your physician if your planned form of exercise is safe and appropriate for you. Also be sure to ask what, if any, adjustments you need to make to your planned exercise program and if and when your exercise routine should be adjusted throughout the duration of your pregnancy.

Once you have spoken with your physician and have clearance to become or stay physically active during your pregnancy, you can get started.

## Exercise guidelines during pregnancy

There are some specific guidelines for exercise that you need to keep in mind and adhere to throughout your pregnancy to make sure you aren't putting your health, or the health of your child, at risk. As you begin, and continue, to exercise throughout pregnancy, keep these guidelines in mind:

- ✔ If you are new to exercise and starting to become physically active as a way to improve your health during pregnancy, make sure to start slowly and increase physical activity gradually. Choosing a lower-intensity form of exercise, such as walking or prenatal yoga, may be your best option.

- ✔ Throughout your pregnancy, listen to your body. Be attuned to signs that it may be time to reduce your exercise level. If you feel you need to slow down, you should.

- ✔ Don't overdo it. Never push yourself to the point of exhaustion or breathlessness during exercise. You should always be able to speak at least a few words while exercising. If you can't, lower your intensity level.

- ✔ Make sure you are wearing supportive footwear to decrease foot, lower leg, and back pain and to prevent injury.

✔ Take frequent breaks as needed and make sure you are staying well hydrated. Aim to drink at least 8 ounces for every 15 to 30 minutes of exercise in addition to 64 ounces or more of fluid for the day.

✔ Watch out for weather extremes. On very hot or very cold days, don't attempt to exercise outdoors. If you want, you may exercise indoors, but listen to your body. Especially on very hot and humid days, even indoor exercise may be taxing on your body.

✔ Limit your risk for injury. Joints are more lax during pregnancy, so your injury risk is higher. For that reason, supportive footwear is important, and you should also avoid unstable ground and rocky terrain. Not only should you do these things to avoid injury, but also to prevent your risk of falls.

✔ Avoid any contact sports or any activities where the risk of falls is high, to prevent injury to yourself or your baby.

✔ Resistance training is a great way to maintain and improve strength and tone during pregnancy. Discuss with your physician how much weight is safe for you to lift (generally lifting over 20 pounds is to be avoided). Also avoid lifting weights above your head or performing any weight-training exercises that may strain your lower body muscles.

✔ Throughout the second and third trimesters, avoid exercises that force you to lie flat on your back. This position can restrict blood flow to the uterus.

✔ Always warm up and cool down before and after exercise, throughout and after your pregnancy.

## The benefits of exercise during pregnancy

Regular exercise provides you with health benefits, such as a healthier cardiovascular system, regardless of your age, sex, or pregnancy. Being physically active, such as by walking on a regular basis, throughout pregnancy offers some additional health benefits unique to pregnancy for both you and your unborn baby. If you get started with your walking routine and stick with it for the duration of your pregnancy, you may experience a variety of benefits that inactive mothers do not.

Benefits of regular exercise for moms-to-be include

✔ **Less weight gain during pregnancy:** Studies have found that women who exercise throughout pregnancy may gain seven less pounds than those who are not physically active while still staying within the healthy weight-gain range, meaning you'll have less to lose after delivery.

✔ **Shorter labor and easier delivery:** Staying fit and building core strength along with cardiovascular endurance may make labor and delivery easier. In fact, one study found that among women who delivered vaginally, those who exercised throughout pregnancy experienced two less hours of active labor than those who did not exercise regularly.

✔ **Decreased back pain:** Although as many as two-thirds of pregnant women experience back pain, you can decrease your risk by staying active and improving core strength, especially in the last two trimesters.

✔ **Decreased risk of swollen feet and ankles:** Due to fluid retention during pregnancy and your growing uterus placing increased pressure on your veins, you may experience swelling in your lower body. However, regular exercise can boost circulation, decrease fluid retention, and fight against swelling.

✔ **Lower risk of gestational diabetes and preeclampsia:** Regular exercise during pregnancy has been found to lower the risk of developing gestational diabetes by as much as 27 percent. In addition, *preeclampsia,* which is a condition marked by elevated blood pressure and excess protein in the urine, may also be decreased with regular exercise.

✔ **Decreased constipation:** Elevated levels of the hormone progesterone along with your growing baby can lead to constipation, but staying active along with a balanced diet rich in fiber can help prevent it.

✔ **Improved energy and mood:** Energy levels can plummet during pregnancy, but a brisk walk can boost energy and help get you through the day. In addition, mothers who exercise have been found to have a lower risk of developing postpartum depression and show a more positive body image throughout pregnancy.

✔ **Decreased need for delivery assistance:** Research has found that women who remain physically active throughout pregnancy may be less likely to need forceps, a C-section, or other forms of intervention during delivery.

✔ **Decreased morning sickness:** Extreme morning sickness may make it hard to exercise, but many pregnant women have found that physical activity lessens the queasiness pregnancy can bring about.

✔ **Improved sleep:** Quantity and quality of sleep may be improved during pregnancy when you remain physically active.

✔ **Bouncing back faster after delivery:** Staying physically active during pregnancy can help you to regain strength and energy, along with your pre-baby weight, more quickly than those who are not active.

✔ **Increased chances of being healthier and leaner in the future:** Research has found that women who exercised throughout pregnancy were more likely to weigh less, have healthier cholesterol levels, and have lower heart rates 20 years after the birth of their child when compared to women who were inactive during pregnancy.

In addition to offering many benefits to the mom-to-be, staying physically active throughout pregnancy can be very beneficial to your unborn child. The benefits of exercise during pregnancy for your baby include

✔ **Improved intelligence and IQ:** Some studies have found that children of mothers who exercise during pregnancy may have better memories and score higher on language and intelligence tests.

✔ **Being leaner at birth, reducing the risk of obesity and diabetes in the future:** Mothers who are active during pregnancy and gain the recommended amount of weight are more likely to give birth to leaner babies. Babies with an excessive fat level are more likely to become overweight in childhood. In addition, overweight newborns of mothers with gestational diabetes are more likely to develop type 2 diabetes later in life.

✔ **Improved heart health:** Research has found that developing babies have more efficient hearts in mothers who exercise, and this higher cardiovascular fitness level may last into childhood.

✔ **Increased athletic ability:** In one study, children who were exposed to exercise in utero were found to perform better at sports when compared to their same-aged peers who were born to mothers who did not exercise during pregnancy.

# Walking After the Birth of Your Baby

Congratulations! Your little one has arrived! As a new mom, you are most likely feeling exhausted and overwhelmed. Exercise may be the last thing on your mind; however, getting back to regular physical activity is one of the best things you can do for yourself. Exercise after the birth of your child can help you

✔ Achieve a healthy body weight

✔ Improve your energy levels and quality of sleep (when you can get it!)

✔ Improve your cardiovascular fitness level

✔ Lift mood and fight stress

✔ Increase strength and muscle tone, especially in your core

✔ Set a great example for your child now and for years to come

# Restarting your walking routine

Now that your baby has been born, you may be wondering when it's safe to start back up with your exercise routine. Although old recommendations used to be to wait six weeks before starting any form of exercise, most healthcare providers now feel that if you've had an uncomplicated vaginal delivery, you may safely begin exercising again as soon as you feel ready.

However, if you've had a Caesarean section, a complicated delivery, or needed extensive vaginal repair, speak with your physician first. You may need to wait six weeks or, in some cases, a little longer, before starting back up with exercise.

Even if you are not yet cleared for exercise, speak to your physician about slowly increasing your overall daily movement. Using a tool such as a pedometer to track your activity can be a great way to help you slowly build back up your daily steps, as you feel comfortable and as medically appropriate, until you are able to jump back into a regular exercise routine.

# Selecting the right intensity for your walking routine

Just as you eased slowly into exercise during pregnancy, you want to do the same after delivery as well. Your body is recovering from a major event and needs time to heal and adjust. If you rush into intense exercise too quickly, you may increase your risk of injury and slow your body's ability to heal and recover from childbirth.

As you plan to get restarted with your walking routine, write down what your goals are for your exercise plan. Is your aim to get back to walking six days per week for one hour? If so, start out by walking every other day. As you walk, start with a slow pace and walk for only 15 to 20 minutes to see how you feel. Increase the duration of your walk every few days until you can comfortably get back to walking for 60 minutes. And give yourself permission to walk more slowly at first. After a few weeks, you can push yourself to walk more quickly and get back to your pre-baby speed once again.

Listen to your body. If you feel very fatigued, are short of breath, or experience any pain, stop exercising and rest. Discuss these symptoms with your physician and see whether an adjustment in your exercise plan is needed. Breaking your walk into intervals throughout the day, such as three 20-minute walks versus one 60-minute walk may also be a more manageable way to exercise at first. Remember, not only is your body adjusting to post-birth movement, but you are also adjusting to becoming a parent. Allow yourself to adjust slowly; don't rush. You'll be able to get back into your old fitness routine before you know it.

## Fitting in walking with a new baby

Now that your baby has arrived, you may be anxious to get back to your pre-baby body as soon as possible. However, you have to take into consideration that life has changed. You now have a tiny person you are responsible for who has many needs and can be quite demanding. More than likely you are sleep deprived, exhausted, and emotional as your body adjusts to the hormone shifts after childbirth.

Finding the time and energy to exercise may seem impossible at first. And that's okay. Give yourself permission, especially in the first few weeks after your baby is born, to just enjoy being a new parent and spending time with your little one. At first, try focusing on just slowly increasing your day-to-day physical activity. Get in a few extra steps here and there. Walk up and down the stairs one extra time. These little bits of activity here and there will start to add up. Use a tool, such as a pedometer, to track and increase your daily steps.

After you feel a bit more comfortable with your new role as a parent and have a bit more energy, you can start to think about fitting in some structured exercise. When you feel ready, talk to your physician and make sure you are cleared to begin exercising. Then get started, but ease into it. Think of ways you can start to increase your daily walking with your baby. If the weather is nice and your pediatrician approves, taking your baby outdoors for fresh air can be a great way to bond. Stroller walks are not only a great way to spend time with your little one, but the added resistance of the stroller intensifies your workout.

If the weather isn't cooperating, you can walk indoors. If you feel comfortable, baby-wearing can be a wonderful bonding experience. Using a baby carrier, you can walk around your home, outdoors, or anywhere you may need to go, such as to the grocery store. Just as with the stroller, wearing your baby adds extra resistance to your walk, increasing the intensity as well as the calorie burn.

# Gathering the Tools You Need to Walk with Baby

As a new mom, you'll most often find that in order to walk, you'll need to bring your baby with you. Although a spouse, partner, family member, or babysitter may be able to watch your newborn at times, planning ways to walk with baby in tow is the wisest way to ensure you'll be able to walk on a regular basis.

When it comes to walking with your baby, there are many aspects you need to take into consideration. First, think of your child's temperament. Is your child one who falls asleep to movement, such as the rocking of a stroller, or does he demand to be held and close to you? What is the weather currently like? If it's very hot or very cold, you'll most likely need to find ways to increase your activity level indoors instead of outside until the temperature is more moderate. Is your child only a few weeks old, or is she months old when you start walking? Your pediatrician may recommend that a newborn who has yet to be vaccinated should not frequently be in public places unless necessary, whereas an older infant may be fine to walk with you in places such as a shopping center or a busy park.

Determine where, when, and how often you will walk. Once you have decided these factors, you can plan how you will walk with your baby. Will you use a stroller to walk your baby or will you wear your baby in a carrier as you walk? Will a loved one watch your baby as you go off to exercise on your own? The answers to these questions will help you determine the best equipment to have on hand for your walking workout post-baby.

## The best equipment for walking with baby

When walking with your baby, two main essentials you want to have are a versatile stroller and a baby carrier that fit your needs and your child's. There are so many strollers and carriers on the market that, as a new parent, you may feel completely overwhelmed. In order to help you make the best choice for your needs, I outline the various features to consider in this section.

When considering the equipment you need for walking with your baby, think about these things:

- Your budget
- Ease of use

✔ How easy the product is to transport if you need to travel with it

✔ Durability and safety

✔ Whether the product will grow with your child

When it comes to selecting a stroller, finding one that is lightweight, easy to open and close, and easy to maneuver is key for many mothers, including myself. There are so many fitness strollers on the market. Some are made for jogging, while others are made for walking on varied terrain. Likewise with baby carriers — there are so many to choose from, you may not know where to start. However, it's important to note that some baby carriers are used only for infants up to a certain weight, whereas others can be adjusted for older, larger infants and toddlers. Some carriers are not appropriate for newborns, so it's important to do your research and select the best option for you.

My personal favorites in these categories are Baby Jogger strollers, due to their ease of use and versatility, and the Lillebaby carrier, due to its back support, varied carrying positions, and ability to be used with newborns through toddlers. Both of these products can be found at many online stores, including www.diapers.com and www.wayfair.com. I offer a detailed comparison list on my website at www.erinpalinski-author.com as well.

## Selecting a baby stroller

Selecting a baby stroller may seem overwhelming, but once you understand the various types and what each offers, it's much easier to make the best choice for you and your baby. Six types of strollers make up the majority available on the market today:

✔ **Standard size:** This is the most common form of stroller and features adequate storage, comfortable seats, and larger wheels. This size stroller is usually built for babies weighing between 16 and 32 pounds. For smaller babies, these strollers often offer a car seat adapter, so the car seat can be placed into the stroller, providing a safe seat for a newborn. A few choices in this category also recline fully flat or offer additional bassinets for newborns. Within this category, you can find strollers with three or four wheels (three wheels tend to lead to better maneuverability) as well as wheels and tires that are meant for all terrains and some that are meant for only flat, smooth surfaces. Make sure you think about where and when you plan to walk to select the best stroller for you.

- **Car seat frame:** These strollers provide a frame that allows a car seat to essentially click into them, converting the car seat into a stroller quickly and easily. Because these frames are inexpensive and compact, not to mention lightweight, they can be great for newborns and through the first year.

- **Lightweight (umbrella):** These strollers are great for travel as they are compact and lightweight. However, they can't be used for babies under 6 months of age and don't offer car seat adapters. Because they have small wheels, they can be difficult to maneuver and are not easy to push on rough surfaces or uneven terrain. These strollers are best suited for older babies who have very good head control and can sit up on their own.

- **Jogging:** If you plan to jog or run with your baby, these strollers are made for you. They typically provide three wheels that are air-filled and have shock absorbers, making them easy to maneuver and appropriate for difficult terrain. These strollers, however, tend to be large and heavy and are not appropriate for babies under 6 months of age.

- **Double:** if you have twins or have an older child as well as a newborn, a double stroller may be the perfect option as it offers two seats either side by side or in tandem. Although narrow enough to fit through most doorways, these strollers are large and can weigh between 21 and 36 pounds.

- **Travel systems:** This is a bundled package that combines a car seat with a stroller. If you choose such a bundle, make sure you are satisfied with the safety of both the car seat and stroller first instead of buying for the convenience factor, or you may end up purchasing additional equipment later on.

Taking note of all the various types of strollers on the market, you may feel you need to purchase multiple options. But if you research each, try them out when you can, and really think about when and where you are walking the most, you can usually narrow down the options to find the best stroller for you. If you will be walking, even power walking, a standard stroller may work great for you, especially if you select one with good maneuverability and all-terrain tires. In addition, if you'll be walking right after your baby is born, make sure you consider a stroller that accommodates newborns, such as one with a car seat adapter, so you can use it now and your baby can grow into it in the future as well.

## Selecting a baby carrier

Baby-wearing has many great benefits for both the mother and the baby; however, you have to make sure to do it correctly for your own safety as well as that of your baby.

Especially during the first six months — and beyond — infants love the snug hold of being close to your chest and find being worn very relaxing. In fact, if you have a fussy infant, this can be a great way to calm her and get her to nap. Even older babies love to be worn as different carrying positions allow them to be worn facing out to the world as well as riding on your back.

When selecting a baby carrier, you must consider your child's age, weight, and the desired use of the carrier. When wearing your baby, you can typically walk to perform common tasks, enjoy a leisurely stroll, or even take a moderate-paced walk, but very fast power walking is not recommended while wearing your baby. However, just the act of wearing your baby increases the intensity of any walk that you perform because you're carrying additional weight. If you want to challenge yourself further, look at adding an incline while walking to intensify your walk. However, while wearing your baby, make sure to stay on even terrain and watch where you are walking to protect against falls.

A large selection of carriers is available on the market:

- **Slings:** For smaller babies, slings can be a great way to keep your baby close, and if you're breastfeeding, to do so discreetly in public. Because slings tend to place all the weight of your baby over one shoulder, they're best for small newborns and infants. Slings typically don't make the best choice for long walks or for hands-free carrying for long periods of time due to the strain you may feel on your shoulder and back.

- **Wraps:** Wraps allow you to evenly distribute your baby's weight across your shoulders and back for more comfortable carrying. Wraps can be worn for extended periods of time without a large amount of muscle fatigue. Many wraps offer various carrying positions depending on the size and age of your child. Depending on the wrap and the carrying position, adequate head and neck support may not be available for newborns.

- **Structured carriers:** Soft, structured carriers typically provide a variety of carrying positions for very young children through toddlers. Depending on the brand you choose, a small carrier may hold only up to a certain size baby and be appropriate for newborns through 4 months; larger carriers may require an additional purchase of a newborn insert for very young babies to provide adequate head and neck support.

When purchasing a baby carrier, think of it like you would a stroller, as a long-term investment. You want to select a carrier that you can use daily and that will grow with your child. For that reason, finding a carrier that provides a versatility of carrying positions is essential. A carrier that can work by providing comfortable carrying for you and your child from newborn through toddlerhood is the ideal carrier.

## *Additional walking must-haves with baby*

As a new parent, you are probably learning to always plan ahead. If you plan to walk with your baby, make sure to bring with you everything you and your baby may possibly need. Make sure your diaper bag is packed with essentials such as diapers, wipes, a changing pad, extra bottles, milk, finger food (for older babies), toys to entertain your baby, a cellphone in case you need to make an emergency call, and, of course, water for yourself to stay hydrated.

When you first start walking with your baby, don't go too far until you see how your baby adjusts to the walk. Some babies love to go for walks or fall asleep instantly from the motion. Others may cry for the whole walk, forcing you to return home shortly after starting. Once you know how your baby typically responds to a walk, you can better plan for what you do and don't need.

# *Tailoring Your Workout as Your Baby Grows*

Getting back into exercise after the birth of your baby is just the start. At first, the biggest struggle is just finding the energy or the time to fit in a few minutes of exercise here and there. As your baby grows and you adjust to becoming a parent, your exercise needs may change as well.

During the first few months after your baby is born, you may be trying to fit in walking to help boost your energy levels, decrease stress, and return to your pre-pregnancy weight. Once you have adjusted to small amounts of exercise, you may want to adjust your walking workout to increase strength and stamina as well as fine-tune your workout to return to your pre-baby body.

Knowing how to recognize the signs that it's time to adjust your workout after your baby has been born is important in helping you to achieve your long-term goals. Speaking of goals, it's important that you set realistic goals for yourself. Getting back to your pre-pregnancy body or regaining your strength within a month of giving birth isn't always realistic. Identifying realistic goals and creating an action plan to achieve them are key to being able to accomplish your goals and maintain your results.

# Identifying the right time to adjust your workout

The first few weeks, and even months, after your baby is born, you may just feel as though you are in "survival mode." Your day revolves around making sure your baby is fed, clean, and rested, and your focus is on his every need. You may not even be thinking about yourself and taking the time to catch up on your own much-needed rest. With limited energy and sleep deprivation, exercise may be the last thing on your mind. However, even small bouts of walking here and there can help you to sleep more restfully (when you get the chance to sleep), boost your mood, and help you to return more quickly to your pre-pregnancy weight.

However, after those first few weeks and months, once you and your baby have established a more regular routine, you may desire to change your exercise routine. Instead of focusing on just trying to increase daily physical activity, you may now want to work on increasing strength, stamina, and speed as well as exercising more consistently to get back to your goal weight. Although your time for exercise may still feel limited as the majority of it may be devoted to caring for your baby, adjusting the ways you walk *with* your baby can help you reach your fitness goals as well as provide a bonding experience with your child.

## Adding resistance

As you feel ready, and after your physician clears you for regular exercise, you can start to look at ways to increase the intensity of your walking workout with your baby. One of the best ways to increase your calorie expenditure while you walk is by adding resistance to your walk. Incorporating your baby into your walking workout helps with this while preventing any guilt you may feel from exercise taking time away from the time you can spend with your baby.

You can add resistance to your walking workout in one of two ways. Using a walking stroller, you can push your child while walking to increase the resistance of your walk. Wearing your child while walking takes the idea of adding resistance up a notch, as you are carrying the full weight of your child with each step, further maximizing the amount of calories you burn.

## Increasing intensity

As you adjust to walking with a stroller or while wearing your child, you can intensify your walking working even further in a few easy ways. As you walk, you can choose to increase the incline of your walk, such as by pushing your stroller uphill or walking up a hill or up stairs while baby-wearing. While walking with a stroller, you can incorporate resistance exercises such as lunges, as shown in Figure 15-1.

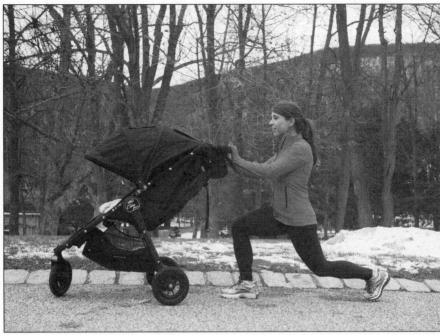

**Figure 15-1:** Walking stroller lunges.

*Photo by Kristen Rath Photography*

To perform lunges, while standing still, hold onto the stroller handle with both hands while keeping your chest raised and your back straight. Step back with your left leg. Slowly bend your front knee, lowering your body closer to the ground. As your front knee bends, your back knee should also bend. Lower your front knee to create a 90-degree angle, making sure that your knee does not pass over your toe line. Slowly rise back up to a stand. Switch legs, and repeat.

While baby wearing, you can use your baby as a form of added weight to perform lower body resistance exercises, such as calf raises and squats as shown in Figures 15-2 and 15-3. Of course, at all times, make sure you are maintaining proper form as you perform these exercises and only do what feels comfortable for you and your baby.

Here's how to perform calf raises: While wearing your baby in a baby carrier facing either inward toward your chest or outward, but centered on your body, stand with legs and feet shoulder width apart. Slowly rise up on the balls of your feet, bringing your heels off the ground. Hold this position for one second, then slowly lower your heels back down. Repeat.

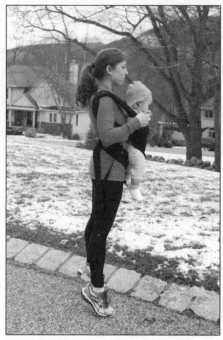

**Figure 15-2:**
Baby-
wearing
calf raises.

*Photo by Kristen Rath Photography*

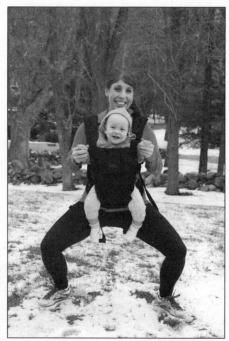

**Figure 15-3:**
Baby-
wearing
squats.

*Photo by Kristen Rath Photography*

To perform squats, follow these instructions: While wearing your baby in a baby carrier facing either inward toward your chest or outward, but centered on your body, stand with your legs shoulder width apart and your toes turned out slightly. Slowly bend your knees to lower your body as if you were sitting in a chair. Make sure to keep your chest upright and don't allow your knees to pass over your toe line. Slowly rise back up by straightening your knees to the starting position; then repeat.

## Setting realistic goals

As a new mother, you're most likely anxious to return to your pre-baby body as quickly as possible. But it's important to be realistic in your goals. You were pregnant for 40 weeks. That's 40 weeks of growth, change, and adjustment for your body. Then there was the trauma of childbirth on your body as well. All of these changes led to the creation of a beautiful child whom you will forever cherish. But, as with any new mother, as grateful as you feel for your amazing child, you also can't wait to be able to zip your skinny jeans back up.

Although it is possible to return to your pre-baby weight, it's important to be patient as well. Even if you get back to your pre-baby weight quickly, you may find that your body is slightly different than it once was. It can take time to build back core strength and re-tone and tighten muscles. And it's important to understand that this process can take time. Just as your baby didn't grow and develop into a healthy newborn overnight, your body won't transform back to its old self overnight either.

Allow yourself time to adjust as a parent and focus on living a healthy lifestyle for yourself and your child. Take it one day at a time. Aim to be a bit more active each day than you were the day before. As you feel up to it and are medically allowed, add a bit of resistance training to your walking workout and work to increase the speed and intensity of each walk. It's great to have weight-loss goals, but keep them small. Losing from ½ to 1 pound a week is a great, and healthy, postpregnancy weight-loss goal. Losing weight too quickly, especially if you are breastfeeding, can impact your milk supply and your body's ability to heal and recover.

As you adjust to your new life as a parent, focus on eating a balanced diet full of whole, unprocessed foods, increasing your daily steps, and adding structured exercise when you feel ready, at least a few times per week. As you follow these guidelines, your weight and measurements will slowly start to return to what they were before. And as they do, you can take comfort in knowing that not only did you lose weight in a healthy way, but it's more likely to stay off for good as well.

# Chapter 16

# Walking with Arthritis and Osteoporosis

...............................................................................

## In This Chapter

▶ Understanding how walking can benefit your joints

▶ Determining how walking can strengthen your bones

▶ Adapting your walking workout for healthy bones and joints

▶ Seeing how weight management fits into the equation

...............................................................................

*I*f you suffer from arthritis or have been diagnosed with osteoporosis, you may feel as though you can't be active without pain or without risk of damaging your joints and bones.

But the truth is that regular walking can actually help you better manage these conditions and decrease pain, and may even help strengthen bones. The fact is, if you suffer from osteoporosis or arthritis, you can't afford not to walk!

If you wake up with chronic joint pain daily, it can be hard to talk yourself into walking. In the same regard, if you have an increased fear of falling that may result in a bone fracture, the idea of becoming more physically active can be frightening.

However, when done correctly, walking for exercise can improve your overall health and even decrease the impact both of these conditions have on your body. Throughout this chapter, I discuss each of these conditions in greater detail and show you how you can safely walk, even with either diagnosis, and gain great health benefits from doing so.

# The Link Between Walking and Arthritis

When it comes to arthritis, there are various forms you may suffer from. Some individuals have osteoarthritis, which is the most common form of arthritis. *Osteoarthritis* is a disease of the entire joint, involving the ligaments, cartilage, joint lining, and underlying bone. As these tissues break down, pain and stiffness increase. Typically, this disease comes on gradually in those over the age of 40. Although there is no cure for osteoarthritis, it can be managed through weight control, exercise, physical therapy, medications, and joint replacement surgery when warranted.

Other individuals have *rheumatoid arthritis* (RA), a chronic, inflammatory disorder that typically impacts the small joints in the hands and feet. Unlike osteoarthritis, which can be brought upon by wear-and-tear damage to joints, RA impacts the linking of the joints, which leads to swelling that can cause pain, bone erosion, and even joint deformity. This disease is considered an autoimmune disorder, whereby the body attacks its own healthy tissue. In some individuals, RA can damage the skin, eyes, lungs, and blood vessels as well. Although this condition can occur at any age, it typically starts after age 40 and is more common in women than in men.

Although the cause of arthritis is not always clear, what is known is that inactivity, weight gain, and an unhealthy diet including inflammatory-rich foods can worsen symptoms. This scenario in turn leads to more pain and less ability to be active, which then results in additional weight gain — a terrible cycle you want to avoid. Of course you should speak with your physician first, but if you are cleared for physical activity, walking, even in small amounts, can help to decrease fatigue, increase strength and flexibility, and improve your quality of life.

## The impact of walking on arthritis outcomes

If you are looking to lose weight, decrease joint pain, and increase your mobility, walking may be the perfect exercise for you. If you are concerned that increasing physical activity may increase joint pain and stiffness, rest assured — the result is actually the complete opposite!

The less exercise you do, the more stiff and painful your joints may become. Keeping the muscles that surround your joints strong is vital to maintaining support to your bones. When you don't exercise, these muscles weaken, which places a larger amount of stress on the joints. Over time, this can worsen arthritis symptoms and stiffen your joints further.

Walking can offer many benefits to individuals with arthritis. Regular walking can help to

- ✔ Build and maintain bone strength
- ✔ Increase the strength in the muscles surrounding and supporting your joints
- ✔ Improve range of motion
- ✔ Decrease fatigue
- ✔ Improve quality of sleep
- ✔ Help you achieve and maintain a healthy body weight, which also decreases stress on the joints

As you strengthen your muscles, increase mobility, and fight off fatigue and stiffness, your joint pain may begin to subside. In fact, one study found that when arthritis sufferers performed low-intensity exercise, such as walking, on a regular basis over a period of six months, they experienced as much as 25 percent less pain and 16 percent less stiffness in their joints. Those are tremendous improvements with just a little bit of walking!

## Is walking right for you?

Any time you have a medical condition, you should always consult your physician before starting or changing any exercise routine. So if you have been diagnosed with arthritis, or suspect it, talk to your doctor first about starting a walking routine and work together to outline a plan that's appropriate for your individual needs.

Depending on the type of arthritis you have, what joints are impacted, and the severity of your symptoms, some exercises may not be appropriate for you. Your doctor and/or physical therapist can help discuss your condition with you and what types of walking will be most beneficial as well as what forms may need to be avoided. For example, if you have arthritis in your knees, walking up stairs repeatedly for exercise or incorporating lunges as a form of resistance training may not be recommended. However incline walking on an even surface may still be an appropriate way to intensify your workout. Your healthcare team can help you determine your individual needs and create a plan that will give you the most health benefits, while preventing the most aggravation of your joints.

Keep in mind that with arthritis, your condition can change over time. You may need to adjust your walking workout during times when pain is increased (such as on very humid or very cold days). You may also need to change your program if your joints worsen over time. Making sure to schedule regular visits with your healthcare team to discuss the progression of your condition and any adjustments that need to be made in your exercise routine is the best way to keep you walking safely and as pain free as possible.

# Improving Joint Health

When it comes to joint health, the more active you can be on a regular basis, the better. In order to stay healthy, joints require motion. When you are inactive for long periods of time, joints, especially those impacted by arthritis, can stiffen. This in turn leads to the weakening of the tissue adjoining the joint. Being physically active at any age can help improve joint health. In fact, research even suggests that regular physical activity in childhood can help to fight against chronic pain in the future.

As you age, muscle strength begins to decline. And the less active you are, the more rapidly this decline occurs. However, at any age, if you start to increase physical activity, you can regain some of this lost strength. By having stronger muscles surrounding your joints, you can help to protect the joints from damage, in turn helping to prevent arthritis or offset some of its symptoms. Many individuals with arthritis who incorporate a low-impact exercise, such as walking, into their regular routine report having less disability and pain. In addition, these same individuals have been found to be able to remain independent longer than similar-aged peers and even perform tasks such as common chores easier and with much less discomfort.

The more you can walk, and the more often, the better you may feel today and long term as well. However, always make sure to speak to your physician first to determine what forms of exercise, and how much, are appropriate for your individual needs.

One strategy that works very well for many individuals with arthritis is walking in intervals throughout the day. If you experience pain and stiffness, trying to walk for 30 minutes at once may be too much on your body. However, if you are able to walk for 10 minutes three times per day, you gain the same health and weight-loss benefits, but the exercise itself becomes more doable.

## Reducing inflammation

You may have heard of the term *inflammation,* but maybe you're not quite sure what it means. Inflammation is essentially an immune response to fight off any infection. With inflammation, the body's white blood cells and the substances they produce are typically activated to fight off an infection from foreign organisms, such as a bacteria or a virus. However, in the case of certain diseases, such as arthritis, the body's immune system triggers an inflammatory response when it mistakenly suspects foreign organisms are present. This is what's known as an *autoimmune* disease, where the body attacks its own healthy tissue as if it were an invader to the body.

Rheumatoid arthritis is an example of an autoimmune disorder, where the body is actually the cause of the inflammation that leads to damage in the joints. Osteoarthritis, on the other hand, is not considered an autoimmune disease, although inflammation is still present in this condition as the joints and surrounding areas become damaged and break down. When inflammation occurs, joint pain, stiffness, and loss of function can result. Decreasing inflammation can help to combat this, and therefore help to manage the symptoms of arthritis.

One way to help decrease inflammation is with low-impact exercise, like walking. One of the greatest benefits of walking is that it's the most basic form of exercise. It's something you already do every day and can just work on doing more often. Because your body is already comfortable with the movement of walking, walking for exercise helps to prevent further stress on your body and joints.

As you walk, circulation in the body is improved. An increase in circulation of blood through the body decreases inflammation around your joints by assisting in moving inflammation out of the joint region. In addition, improved circulation increases the rate at which blood, oxygen, and nutrients are brought to your joints, promoting healing. All of these things improve the overall health of your joint and how it functions, lessening pain and stiffness.

In combination with exercise, eating a diet consisting of mainly whole foods and limiting processed foods, simple sugars, and saturated fats can also aid in lessening inflammation. Compression garments, such as the Breg Silicone Elastic Ankle Support Wrap, may also provide some relief.

# *Walking and mobility*

Have you ever heard the phrase "if you don't use it, you lose it"? This axiom could never be truer than it is for physical activity. As you age, you begin to lose muscle mass and experience a decline in muscle strength. However, staying physically active on a regular basis helps to fight against this muscle loss and keep all the muscles in your body stronger. When muscles are strong, they are better able to support your bones and joints. Weak muscles lead to increased strain and pressure on bones and joints, which can negatively impact them over time and increase inflammation. Keeping your muscles strong by walking on a regular basis can help you prevent this.

In addition to strengthening muscles, walking also helps to move your joints through their full range of motion. As you take a step, your hips are stretched, your knees and ankles bend, your shoulders pump your arms, and so on. By helping to move your joints through their full range of motion repeatedly, you can increase your overall flexibility. The more flexible your joints are, the less risk of injury you have. In addition, increased flexibility reduces joint and muscle stiffness, which helps to further increase mobility.

When it comes to improving mobility, the more you can move, and the more often, the better. But remember to take it slow. If your joints are painful and stiff right now, and even standing feels like a struggle, just aim to walk a few minutes a day at first. Once you start to feel like you have a bit more strength and range of motion, increase to 10 minutes per day, then 15, and so on. Don't overdo it and push to walk too much too fast, or you'll increase the risk of burning out or injuring yourself. Slow and steady is the best way to be able to walk regularly over time.

# Walking to Fight Osteoporosis

*Osteoporosis* is a disease in which bones become so weak and brittle that even a minor fall, or a stress like coughing, can lead to a fracture. Bone, which is living tissue, is constantly being absorbed and replaced in your body. When the body can't keep up with the creation of new bone to replace old bone, osteoporosis develops. Fractures of the hip, wrist, and spine are the most common ones caused by this disease; however, fractures can happen in any bone in the body. Men and women of any age and race can be impacted by this disease; however, white or Asian women, especially those past menopause, are at the greatest risk.

Osteoporosis is a widespread problem and many individuals may not even realize they are at risk until they suffer a fracture. Annually worldwide, osteoporosis causes more than 8.9 million fractures. In addition, it is estimated that 1 in 3 women over age 50 will experience osteoporotic fractures, as will 1 in 5 men over age 50 at some time in their life. And, while you may not think of osteoporosis as a serious medical condition, in women over 45 years of age, osteoporosis accounts for more days spent in the hospital than many other diseases, including diabetes, myocardial infarction, and breast cancer.

A healthy diet, especially one providing an adequate amount of vitamin D and calcium, is essential for healthy bones. However, even more importantly, regular weight-bearing exercise, such as walking, is needed to stress and strengthen bones, protecting against this disease.

# The impact of walking on osteoporosis outcomes

Regular exercise is vital in preventing and slowing the progression of osteoporosis. In addition, regular exercise can help to increase balance and coordination, reducing the risk of falls. Falls are one of the leading causes of fractures and death in individuals over the age of 65. The range of motion, strength, flexibility, or coordination regular exercise helps you to build and maintain can decrease your fall risk, helping to further protect you from fractures.

*Weight-bearing exercise,* or exercise in which you support your own body weight (such as walking where your body weight is supported by your feet and legs) is very beneficial for bone health at any age, but especially for those at an older age with an increased risk of osteoporosis. As you perform weight-bearing exercise, tension is applied to the muscle and the bone. The body then responds to this stress by increasing the density of your bones. In younger individuals, an increase in bone density of as much as 2–8 percent can be seen each year with regular exercise. This potential makes becoming active at a young age and staying active critical for long-term bone health.

Walking alone provides weight-bearing exercise for your lower body. However, you can also increase strength and bone density in your upper body as you walk by using *walking weights* or dumbbells. These weights come wrapped in neoprene with straps for your hands, making them easy to carry for the duration of your walk. One brand I like to use is Gold's Gym 2-pound Soft Walking Weights, which can be found at retailers such as Sports Authority, Walmart, and www.wayfair.com.

You can also use resistance bands during your walk to increase strength and muscle mass, and improve bone density. These bands, similar to rubber bands, provide resistance as you stretch them, but they're lightweight, making them easy to carry and transport. You can replicate almost any dumbbell exercise with resistance bands. These bands can be found at many sporting goods stores or online retailers. One brand I recommend is the TheraBand Resistance Band Loops, which can be purchased at retailers such as www.wayfair.com. They come in different weights, or tightness. Start with the lower weight and work up to tighter bands as your muscles strengthen.

Research has shown that long, brisk walks can improve bone density and mobility. In fact, one study found that older women who walked for just four hours per week were able to reduce their risk of hip fracture by over 40 percent. So as you can see, just a small amount of walking can lead to healthier bones lifelong.

# Determining whether walking is appropriate if you have osteoporosis

If you've been diagnosed with osteoporosis, starting an exercise program may seem a bit scary. You may be apprehensive, feeling as though exercising may increase your risk of falls and fractures. You may think that by playing it safe and staying sedentary, you can avoid osteoporosis-related fractures.

But the less active you are, the more bone you lose more rapidly. Even bending over or coughing can cause a fracture with severe osteoporosis, and those are things you can't avoid. Instead of letting the fear of falling hold you back, find out how to safely exercise so you can improve your bone health and prevent further bone loss.

Walking on a regular basis provides your body, especially your lower body, with weight-bearing exercise as it carries your upper body for the duration of the walk. Walking helps to strengthen the spine along with the bones throughout your lower body. Additional resistance training can be beneficial in further strengthening your bones. Incorporating Total Body Workout Walking and Resistance Walking into your walking program (see Chapter 10 for details) can help to further strengthen bones and decrease fracture risk. Of course, before starting or changing any exercise program, discuss doing so with your physician to see what forms of exercise would be the most beneficial for your individual health needs.

As you get started with a walking program, you want to decrease your risk of falls — and therefore fractures — as much as possible. Being mindful of where and how you walk can help. Make sure you walk with correct form and posture. Keeping your chest upright, shoulders back, core tight, and eyes looking in front of you instead of down can help to maintain good balance and decrease fall risk. If you choose to walk outdoors, make sure to walk on even surfaces. Look out for bumps, cracks in the sidewalk, uneven terrain, or slick or icy conditions, which can cause you to lose your balance and fall. Carrying a walking stick can be a great way to improve your balance and prevent a fall as well.

If you choose to walk indoors, just as with walking outdoors, keep an eye out for any surfaces that can increase fall risk. Avoid uneven floors, cracks in floor surfaces, and slippery surfaces such as a wet floor to prevent a fall. If you walk on a treadmill, make sure you walk at a comfortable pace and are familiar with the emergency shutoff on the machine, so you can stop if needed.

# Planning Your Walking Routine with Arthritis

Walking offers many benefits to the management and treatment of arthritis. From decreasing joint pain and stiffness to improving body weight and increasing range of motion, walking on a regular basis can do a lot to improve your quality of life with arthritis. However, you may be wondering just how to get started.

If you are currently living with a large amount of pain or stiffness, trying to take even a few steps may seem unmanageable. But when it comes to arthritis, the more you can start moving and keep moving, the better off you'll feel. One of the best ways to get started with walking is to use a simple tool such as a pedometer and just focus on increasing the number of steps you take each day. Wear a pedometer on your waistband for three days just to get your average number of daily steps. Then try adding just 100 to 200 extra steps per day to get started.

For example, say you walk 2,000 steps per day on average. For the next few days, aim to walk 2,100 steps. When that feels comfortable, build up to 2,200 steps, and so on. As you build up to walking more and more steps, you may start to feel a decrease in stiffness and pain, making it easier to add more steps over time. Remember, when it comes to exercise, every little bit, no matter how small, makes a difference in improving your health.

The key to walking with arthritis is to avoid joint pain from swelling and inflammation. You can relieve short-term joint pain with a few simple techniques at home, including *capsaicin,* a substance found in chili peppers that may relieve joint pain from arthritis and other conditions. Capsaicin blocks substance P, which helps transmit pain signals, and it triggers the release of chemicals in the body called endorphins, which block pain. Side effects of capsaicin cream include burning or stinging in the area where it's applied. Another topical option is an arthritis cream containing the ingredient *methyl salicylate,* found in Bengay, which is available at any drugstore. Braces and wraps also help, such as the FLA Therall Joint Warming Knee Support, which can be purchased at medical supply companies or online at stores such as Amazon. Always discuss which over-the-counter creams and braces are most appropriate for you with your physician before using.

# Taking precautions with arthritis

If you have arthritis, it's important to take a few extra precautions when walking to protect your joints against any injury or further damage:

- ✔ Choose flat, even surfaces, especially if you have joint issues in your hips, knees, or feet, to decrease the stress and impact on these joints.

- ✔ Choose supportive footwear. You may want to speak to your physician or podiatrist about shoe inserts that can add an extra layer of shock absorption to reduce stress and pressure on your joints.

- ✔ If you start to experience pain while walking, stop and rest. Don't ignore pain or push through it, which can lead to injury. Rest and continue when the pain has lessened. If pain continues or worsens, contact your physician.

- ✔ Maintain good posture and body alignment throughout your walk. Not only can this protect against falls, but keeping your body in the proper position helps to strengthen your muscles and takes pressure off your joints.

- ✔ Watch the timing of your pain medications. Try to avoid taking them before exercise, as they may mask pain you may experience from exercise. Discuss the appropriate timing of these medications in relationship to walking with your physician.

You know your body best. Listen to it. If you feel an increase in pain or discomfort while walking, decrease your intensity or rest and continue at a later time. Be mindful of the precautions listed previously so you can continue with your exercise routine on a regular basis while keeping your joints and bones healthy.

# Adapting your workout

How much, how often, and how intensely you choose to walk all depend on your individual fitness level and current condition. If you've already been walking on a regular basis and are looking to increase the intensity of your workout to help you burn more calories and shed pounds, you can certainly do so; however, you need to make a few minor adjustments to avoid worsening your arthritis.

One of the best ways to increase the intensity of your walking workout is to incorporate interval training. With this strategy, you walk at a slower speed for a set period of time (say, five minutes) and then walk at a faster pace for a shorter period of time (say, one minute). You then repeat these intervals over and over again for the duration of your walk. Adding an incline to your walking workout can also increase the intensity. However, if you have arthritis in any of the joints of your lower body or back, this isn't your best option as it may increase the stress on these joints and, in turn, increase your discomfort. Instead, focus on adding interval training on a flat surface to boost your calorie burn.

Light resistance training, either during or after your walk, can also be a great way to increase strength, boost metabolism, and increase your range of motion. The exercises in the Resistance Walking and Total Body Workout Walking plans in Chapter 10 can all be incorporated safely. However, if you have arthritis pain in any joints while performing some of the moves (for example, knee pain with lunges), avoid those particular exercises. You can also speak to your physician or physical therapist about other resistance exercises that may be appropriate for you.

If your arthritis is severe and walking for any length of time causes a large amount of pain, you may want to see whether you can find a location to walk in the water. Walking back and forth as well as side to side in waist-deep water is a great way to burn calories, increase resistance to strengthen muscles, and increase your flexibility, all while decreasing pressure and wear and tear on your joints. Many local YMCAs, gyms, and healthcare facilities have pools and even teach water walking classes you may participate in. Speak to your healthcare provider about braces that may help to provide stability, support, and relief as well. Once you know which brace may be helpful, check out a store such as The Brace Shop (www.braceshop.com), which offers a large selection of hip, knee, ankle, and posture braces.

# Planning Your Walking Workout with Osteoporosis

Getting started with a walking routine if you've been diagnosed with osteoporosis can be nerve-wracking, especially if you're concerned about the risk of falls and fractures. But using your muscles can actually help to protect against fractures and falls. In addition, by taking certain precautions and planning ahead, you can walk safely while building your bone density and helping to prevent your osteoporosis from worsening.

Before getting started with your walking program, make sure you discuss with your physician what forms of exercise are the safest for you and what you should avoid. Make sure you understand which of your bones have been affected by osteoporosis, so you know where your highest risk factors are. Think about where and when you plan to walk so you can assess your walking route and location and pinpoint any areas that may be a high fall risk.

As you plan your routine, think of ways you can increase the resistance throughout your walking workout. For instance, incorporating the Resistance Walking or Total Body Workout Walking plan (refer to Chapter 10) is a great way to help further stress bones (which can help promote the strengthening of bones) and build bones, while also increasing metabolism to help you achieve your goal weight.

## Precautions with osteoporosis

The number-one risk of exercising with osteoporosis is the risk of falling, which can lead to fractures. Making sure that where and how you choose to walk are as free of fall risks as possible is the key to a safe workout. Before you head out to walk, make sure to assess the following items:

- ✔ Where will you be walking? Is the terrain even and free of debris or uneven surfaces that can increase fall risk?

- ✔ Are you wearing supportive footwear that provides good shock absorption as well as rubber soles that protect against slips and falls?

- ✔ If you will be walking outdoors, check the weather before heading out. Is there a possibility of wet or icy surfaces that can increase your chance of slipping?

- ✔ If you will be walking up and down stairs, do the stairs have a handrail you can grab onto if you lose your balance?

- ✔ If you will be walking indoors, is the surface free of slippery spots, cracks, or uneven surfaces that can increase fall risk?

- ✔ Are you practicing correct posture as you walk to help decrease fall risk?

Avoid exercises that cause you to bend and twist, such as sit-ups, toe touches, or certain yoga poses, as they can compress your spine and increase fracture risk. Before starting any exercise routine, show your physician your planned exercise routine, including any planned stretches and resistance exercises, to ensure they are appropriate for you.

## Adapting your workout

Of course, you want to take precautions against any fall risk or anything that may result in a fracture. You may be wary of increasing the intensity of your workout because doing so may increase your fracture risk. However, this isn't necessarily true. You can certainly increase your exercise intensity safely. And doing so can actually benefit your bones.

Adding positive stress to your walking workout, such as briskly walking uphill or walking up stairs is a great way to add an incline to your workout and increase your calorie burn. In addition, these activities further stress your bones, helping to build bone density and prevent osteoporosis from worsening. You can choose to add an incline in a number of ways:

- ✔ **Walk uphill briskly.** Choose an outdoor location that offers a hilly terrain. Just make sure that the hill is free from uneven surfaces or other areas that may increase your fall risk.

- ✔ **Increase your incline on a treadmill.** With a treadmill, you can control your level of incline. Start slowly by adding 1–2 percent incline and build up as you feel comfortable.

- ✔ **Walk up stairs.** Walking up stairs is a great way to boost your heart rate and stress the bones in your lower body, including your hips and spine. However, make sure that you have access to a hand rail.

# Walking and Weight Management for Joint Health

Because you decided to pick up this book, most likely your main goal is to lose weight and keep it off. And though your main reasons for losing weight may be to look better and get back into the clothes you love, maintaining a healthy weight provides many more benefits than just an improved appearance. If you suffer from arthritis, losing weight and keeping it off may be key to decreasing joint pain and increasing your overall mobility.

Body weight plays a major role in the amount of stress placed on your joints. Being just 10 pounds over your ideal weight increases the force on your knee by 30 to 60 pounds with every single step you take. In fact, overweight women have nearly four times the risk of osteoarthritis of the knee, whereas overweight men have five times the risk. These statistics alone show just how much of a negative impact excess weight can have on joint health.

Losing even 10 pounds can make a major impact on the stress placed on your joints and on reducing pain. As pain is reduced, being more physically active on a regular basis is possible, which helps to promote additional weight loss. As you can see, this possible cycle is one that can lead to achieving and maintaining a healthy body weight long term.

Although losing weight can't repair damage that has already occurred to your joints, it can help to slow the progression of osteoarthritis and prevent further joint damage. One study found that when obese men lost enough weight to go from being classified as obese to being classified as overweight, osteoarthritis of the knee decreased by 21.5 percent, and in women, osteo-arthritis decreased by as much as 31 percent. And if you don't already have arthritis, but are worried about developing it, you have even more reason to aim for achieving a healthy body weight. Studies have found that over a ten-year period, losing just 10 pounds may reduce your risk of developing arthritis by more than 50 percent.

# Walking and Weight Management for Bone Health

One of the biggest conundrums when it comes to weight loss is the impact it has on bone health. For most health conditions, losing weight and achieving a healthy body weight can improve your overall health and better manage your disease state. For instance, joint health, blood pressure, and heart health are all improved when weight loss is achieved. However, when you're overweight, carrying the extra poundage actually increases the stress on your bones. When bones are stressed, they strengthen over time. This is why one of the main risk factors for osteoporosis is being of a slight frame or a low body weight.

Although maintaining a higher body weight may help to protect you against osteoporosis, it greatly increases your risk for diseases such as diabetes, heart disease, and even certain cancers. So losing weight and maintaining a healthy body weight should always be a health priority. However, regardless of whether weight is lost for voluntary or involuntary reasons, weight loss, especially later in life, can increase the rate of hip-bone loss and therefore increase the risk of fractures.

To decrease your risk of sustaining a fracture, it's essential to include regular exercise, specifically weight-bearing exercise, as you aim to lose weight. Losing weight through diet only, without any exercise, can accelerate bone loss. However, performing weight-bearing exercise, such as walking, on a regular basis throughout your weight-loss program can help to protect against bone loss and even strengthen bone density over time.

# Chapter 17

# Overcoming Obstacles

* * * * * * * * * * * * * * * * * * * * * * * * * * * * * * * * * * * * *

## In This Chapter

▶ Understanding obstacles that may derail your walking plan

▶ Making time for walking

▶ Finding the motivation to keep going

▶ Preventing injury

* * * * * * * * * * * * * * * * * * * * * * * * * * * * * * * * * * * * *

Maybe you've been walking for a week or two, but now you've run into an unforeseen obstacle. Or maybe you've made it for a month or more already.

No matter how long you've been walking, when you exercise on a regular basis, you're bound to face some obstacles at times. Perhaps your schedule has changed and you're struggling to find the time to fit in your regular walk. Maybe your weight loss has started to slow and you're losing the motivation to continue walking. Or perhaps you've been sidelined with an injury and are now struggling to restart your walking routine.

Whatever the reason for your struggle to keep up with your walking workout and no matter what obstacle you face, you can overcome it and get back on track so that you can achieve your long-term weight-loss goals (and most importantly, maintain your weight loss as well). It may not be easy, but it is doable!

Throughout this chapter, I discuss the most common obstacles that may throw your exercise routine off course. I look at the obstacles in depth and provide some solutions to overcome these challenges and help you stay on track.

Even if you're not yet facing any challenges to walking on a regular basis, you most likely will at some point in time. If you plan ahead for potential obstacles, you can recognize when they may present themselves and have an action plan ready to tackle the challenge and stay on track. The more prepared you are in advance, the less likely an obstacle is to derail your progress.

# Facing Common Obstacles That Can Impact Walking

Any obstacle, no matter how small, can throw you off track when it comes to regular exercising. Missing just one workout may seem like nothing, but it can lead to a pattern of missed workouts, inconsistent exercise, slowed results, frustration, and finally giving up on walking all together. To prevent this from happening, you have to tackle obstacles and challenges head on. Don't let them take control of your schedule and prevent you from walking. If you do, you may slowly, over time and possibly without even realizing it, give these obstacles permission to stop you from exercising all together.

If you've exercised regularly in the past, can you remember why you stopped? Did something happen that made it more difficult to continue with your workout? Did you experience a change in schedule, a life event such as having a baby or changing jobs, or did you just lose motivation? You may not even know why you stopped before. But take a moment and really think about it. Try to remember. It's possible that the same obstacle may derail you again if you don't address it before it becomes an issue.

If you've never exercised regularly before, think about potential challenges that may stop you from continuing. If you push yourself too hard at first and try to walk too much or too quickly, you may injure yourself or burn out, causing you to stop walking for a period of time. If you are new to exercise, you may already be struggling with obstacles such as when to find the time to walk each day or how to stay motivated to continue walking on a regular basis.

Scheduling and motivation, although big challenges, aren't the only obstacles that can cause you to get off track. For instance, what if the weather changes and you can no longer walk outdoors? How can you continue your walking workout with little to no equipment? What if you can only walk indoors, but have a limited budget and can't afford a treadmill or a gym membership? These are real obstacles that anyone can face at any time. However, each of these challenges has solutions. Thinking about these challenges in advance and coming up with solutions that will work for you if you face them helps you stay on track no matter what life throws at you.

## Walking with limited outdoor access

If you started your walking program in the fall or the spring, walking outdoors may have seemed like the perfect idea. The outdoors is accessible everywhere, it's free, and it offers unlimited terrains and views. However, as the weather starts to change and becomes too hot or too cold to continue, you may have to change your plans. When winter arrives, your typical walking path may become covered in snow. In the summer, excessive heat and humidity may make walking outdoors some days unsafe.

If you don't have access to a gym or a treadmill and you can't go outdoors, what can you do? The good news is that you still have lots of options! For starters, you can invest in a simple pedometer like the Sportline or Omron pedometer you can find at www.walmart.com for around $15. Or you can look into the many high-tech gadgets, wearable technology, and apps that track your overall daily activity, like Fitbit, to view your steps, distance, time, calories burned, and even sleep patterns. Put your pedometer on your waistband and set a goal for yourself. Remember that about every 2,000 steps equal 1 mile of walking. So, if you typically walked 2 miles outdoors, set a goal to walk indoors until you rack up 4,000 steps on your pedometer. Walk around your home, up and down your stairs, and back and forth in your hallway or living room. You can also use a treadmill at home — Walmart and www.wayfair.com sell them for $90 and up. If that doesn't seem exciting, head to an indoor shopping mall and walk briskly until you achieve your step goal.

If using a pedometer doesn't excite you, you can buy or rent exercise DVDs that focus on walking (I've listed some of my favorites on my website at www.erinpalinski-author.com) and watch in the comfort of your own home office. Follow along and you can walk 1 or more miles in place! If you do have access to equipment like a treadmill, this is a great time to start using it. Even if you prefer to walk outdoors, during bad weather days (or anytime it may not be safe to head outside), getting on the treadmill can be just as effective as walking outdoors. When walking on the treadmill, you can replicate your outdoor walk by using the incline to replicate hilly terrain and walking the same distance you would if you were outdoors.

## Walking with limited equipment

Although it may seem like you need gadgets, tools, and fancy equipment to successfully walk away the pounds, that's really not true. The only things you need to start walking are supportive footwear and a pair of feet. There's no need to spend large amounts of money or devote a huge chunk of time to preparing for your walk. Just put on your shoes and get going!

If you're looking for ways to keep yourself entertained while walking and don't have access to music or headphones, try walking outdoors. The scenery is always changing and gives you plenty to look at and focus on. Walking indoors in public places, such as shopping centers, is also a great way to keep your attention. People-watching can always be entertaining and help to prevent your walk from becoming boring. You can even carry a portable phone or cellphone and catch up with family and friends as you walk as well.

You don't have to invest money in large, expensive equipment like a treadmill. You can walk anywhere, anytime, such as outside in your neighborhood, at a park, or even at a shopping center. That's the greatest thing about walking — it's so easy to do anywhere and costs little to nothing. Research the best walking areas around you. Where can you easily and safely walk outdoors as well as indoors (on bad weather days)? Then, set up a plan to get to these locations and determine how often you'll go, so you can walk on a regular basis.

## Walking on a budget

So you don't have the money to join the gym or purchase fancy workout equipment for your home — so what? That doesn't have to stop you from walking. Walking is ideal for individuals on a budget because it costs little to nothing to do. All you need is supportive footwear; that's it! Even high-tech socks and shoes are now affordable. The website at www.thewalkingcompany.com is a great place to start; check my site for other suggestions and coupons. Don't get discouraged if your budget is limited for now. You can still successfully walk off the pounds, increase the intensity of your workout when needed, and keep the weight off — all without ever opening your wallet.

Without access to a treadmill or a gym, just head outdoors or to a public indoor walking area, such as a shopping center, to get moving. If you don't have access to a pedometer to track your steps and your distance, don't worry. Instead, map out your own walking route to figure out just how far you are walking (it was done this way in the pre-pedometer era, after all!). If you're walking outside, drive the route with a car and use its odometer to track the distance of your planned route. If you're walking inside, measure out (or even count the steps of) your planned route to determine the distance of one walking lap. For instance, if you plan to walk in your house and know that your hallway is 100 steps long, every time you walk down and back, you'll have covered 200 steps. So if you walk your hallway ten times, you'll have walked 1 mile.

Even without equipment or an accommodating budget, you can intensify your walking workout when you need to. Walk faster or longer, or add interval training to mix up your workout. If you want to add incline, walk up a hill outdoors or walk up and down stairs indoors. You can even perform resistance exercises, such as the ones I outline in Chapter 10, with minimal equipment. You can use your own body weight, or if you want to add weight, look at affordable resistance bands or even use equally weighted water bottles as dumbbell replacements! If you're budget conscious, check websites like www.endomondo.com where you can track your walking and weight loss for free. Also, look for coupons on my site as well as sites such as www.RetailMeNot.com for more ways to save.

# Fitting Walking into Your Schedule

Even if you have all the equipment possible and an unlimited budget, you still may find yourself struggling to stay on track with your exercise routine. Why? Possibly, you're just having difficulty scheduling time in your day to fit it in. No matter who you are or what you do for a living, I'm sure you are quite busy. Between balancing work schedules, family schedules, time for yourself or to visit with friends, appointments, and so on, finding time for exercise can feel almost impossible.

But when it really comes down to it, even if you are the busiest person on the planet, if you really want to exercise, you can make time for it. You may need to be creative and multitask, but you can do it. And I'm here to help you! If you found out tomorrow that you needed to schedule in a very important meeting with your boss, or you needed to take your child to a healthcare professional, you'd find the time to book those appointments, right? Well, what's more important than your own health? Failing to make an appointment with yourself to exercise is the same as skipping an appointment with your doctor, because making time to get active and stay active is key to keeping yourself healthy. There's always the time; you just have to make it. You can even use a free calendar app, like www.google.com/calendar, to schedule your walk as well as get notifications to remind you.

## Walking with a busy schedule

You may have the same schedule day after day, or perhaps your schedule is different every single day. No matter what your schedule is typically like, take out a piece of paper and write out your schedule for tomorrow. Write down every place you will be, how long you'll be there, and what you'll be doing. Now look at your schedule. Is there any downtime? Even five minutes here and there between appointments or maybe a few minutes before your day gets started or after you get home?

Any downtime that you have is time that you can squeeze in a walk. Remember, walking is cumulative. Walking for five minutes between appointments five times during the day is the same as scheduling in a 25-minute walk. Now, maybe your schedule is jampacked: You leave the house at the break of dawn, commute to work, attend nonstop meetings, commute home, have a quick dinner, and go to bed. It doesn't look like there's much time to walk in there, does it? What about those meetings? Are any of them conference calls where you'll be on the phone at your desk rather than in a meeting room? If so, get up and pace during the call instead of sitting. If not, park as far away as possible when you get to work so you can squeeze in additional steps walking back and forth to your car. You can even see your friend's availability on his online calendar and schedule a time to walk together. It's often harder to skip out on a friend than yourself, so planning to walk with a friend is a great motivator or trick to keep yourself on track!

Even if you're running from one meeting or appointment to another day after day, you most likely can still find a few minutes each day to fit in a walk. If you arrive to an appointment early, walk around the parking lot or building until your scheduled appointment time. If you take a bathroom break during the day, walk the long way to and from the bathroom to increase your steps. Even though these small amounts of walking may seem trivial, they really do add up.

## Walking on the job

If you work all day and have no time to get to the gym, don't worry. You can still fit in a decent amount of walking and start shedding pounds with just a small amount of effort. Examine your entire work day and look for any opportunities that may allow you to walk, even if just a few steps. For instance, start when you first come to work in the morning. Park farther away than you normally would, so you can rack up extra steps coming and going from work.

Once inside, think of ways you can fit in additional steps. Can you walk a lap around your place of work once or twice before getting started for the day? Can you do the same before leaving at the end of the day? Do you get any breaks at work? If so, can you use these breaks to walk around your building for a few minutes? How about at lunchtime? If you take a lunch break, can you walk a few minutes before and after eating? If you're on the phone for any length of time while working, can you walk while talking? Even if you sit at a computer all day long, you can still fit in a few extra steps. Try standing at the computer every once in a while instead of sitting throughout the day. For every half hour of work, stand up, stretch your legs, and walk 50–100 steps before sitting back down. Or even look into purchasing a treadmill desk (check out www.trekdesk.com) to help you rack up steps while you work. All of these tiny changes add up to big results when it comes to your health and your weight.

## Walking with your family

Whether you are a stay-at-home parent or a working parent, trying to juggle family commitments and still find time to exercise can be a challenge. However, if you work exercise into family time, you can improve not just your health, but also the health of your entire family. Think of all the things you and your family do together when you have "family time." Do you sit down to watch TV as a family after finishing dinner? Instead, why not take a walk together as a family? You can all catch up on your day while fitting in physical activity.

If you walk at dusk or nighttime, wear clothing with reflectors to keep your family safe. Many retailers, such as Kohls or Under Armour, carry a wide selection. You can also bring headlamps. And, don't forget your dog! Even the dog can wear a dog pedometer if *everyone's* tracking his fitness, and giving children pedometers is a great way to teach them about fitness too. A baby carrier or stroller is a must if you have a family member who's too young to walk; bringing the baby makes it a real family event.

If it's too cold or dark to walk together, think of ways your family can get moving together indoors. Can you play an active game indoors to rack up extra steps? Can you go out together as a family to walk indoors, such as window shopping at a mall together? Even family chores can allow you to increase your daily steps. For instance, vacuuming or cleaning the floors in your home can easily help you to walk an additional 1,000 steps or more. If you have young children at home, chasing after them can also bump up your steps.

When it comes to walking more on your own or as a family, examine your daily routine and think about all the times you are sitting during the day. What are you doing during these times? Think of ways you can adjust the activity so you can stand or walk instead. For example, stand up when typing versus sitting in a chair. Walk during the commercial breaks of your favorite TV show instead of sitting on the couch. Pace while talking on the phone instead of lounging in a chair. The more ways you can find to squeeze in additional steps, the quicker and easier it will be to achieve your weight-loss goals and maintain them long term.

# Staying Motivated with Your Walking Routine

There's one main ingredient to losing weight and keeping it off long term, and that's consistency. However, in order to stay consistent with your walking routine, you need to be motivated to walk. Feeling excited about walking is easy in the beginning. Starting your walking plan is new, and the idea of losing weight and inches quickly pushes you to be consistent day after day for a while. However, over time, as you either become accustomed to your walking workout or your results begin to slow a bit, you may start to feel unmotivated.

Although it's completely normal for your motivation level to change over time and even lessen a bit as your workout routine is no longer new, it's important to be on the lookout for signs of a decrease in motivation so you can address it before it overcomes you and makes sticking with your walking routine a challenge. If you recognize a decrease in motivation right away and work to address it, you can continue to feel challenged and excited about your workout. And when you feel that you are pushing yourself in a good way and look forward to walking each day, it's easy to stay on track with your exercise plan and be consistent. And that consistency is what will ultimately allow you to achieve your long-term weight-loss and health goals.

Keep in mind that motivation can rise and fall throughout your weight-loss journey. Even during the course of just one day, motivation can change. For instance, you may wake up feeling energized and ready to be as physically active as possible, but as soon as you get to work you may become overwhelmed with stress. This stress may lead to a change in mood, increased fatigue, and limited motivation to stick with your planned walk at the end of your workday. Or, you may wake up feeling tired and run down and decide there's no way you'll walk today. But then, you may run into an old friend who has lost weight by walking and inspires you to keep up with your own weight-loss efforts. Another option to keep you motivated may be to look into using comfortable ear buds, headphones, or a Bluetooth earpiece such as Jawbone so you can listen to music or talk while you walk.

Walking with a friend to whom you are accountable, or involving friends and family with your fitness goals, can also help to increase motivation. For instance, using an app like the Fit Friendzy Exercise Challenge allows you to challenge friends to a workout. Or look into using Nike+ GPS maps, which route your walk while tracking your run's distance, pace, time, and burned calories.

If you love social media, motivate yourself by posting the start of your walk to Path or Facebook, and hear real-time cheers through your headphones whenever one of your friends likes or comments on that post. On EveryMove, users earn points from their physical activities that can be redeemed for rewards from brands, their insurance company, and their employers. Even a Fitbit tracker can help you feel motivated. It tracks all your movement during the day, which means you actually see yourself reaching your goals quicker, whereas tracking your daily steps otherwise may be difficult. Check out my website for more useful apps that can motivate you.

Every day is different, and you can't always know ahead of time how you'll feel and what situations may impact your motivation for the day ahead. However, if you plan ahead and have an action plan to keep yourself feeling excited and motivated about your workout, no matter what the day brings, you are more likely to stay on track and achieve your goals long term.

## Understanding why motivation may change

Ask yourself how you feel about your walking plan right now. Are you excited to get started? Do you look forward to your walk each day? Or do you feel as though you are forcing yourself to walk every day even though it's the last thing you really want to do? Be honest with yourself to assess your level of motivation right now. Even if your motivation level is as high as it can be, it's possible that a situation or an event (or even just exercise fatigue from doing the same thing day after day) may cause your motivation to wane over time.

Motivation can start to diminish for many reasons. Some of the biggest reasons include the following:

- ✔ Boredom with your current exercise routine due to repetition of the same exercise day after day
- ✔ Feeling as though you have limited time to fit in exercise
- ✔ Being discouraged with slow or limited weight-loss results
- ✔ Feeling discouraged if health measurements, such as cholesterol or blood pressure levels, remain unchanged even with consistent exercise
- ✔ Lack of support from family and friends

You've most likely experienced at least one or two of these situations before, perhaps with other lifestyle changes you've made, if not with exercise. For example, if you overhauled your diet only to see limited weight loss or feel a lack of support at home, you probably found yourself slowly going back to old habits. Or if your schedule changed or your stress levels increased, the first thing to go out the door may have been your exercise plan as you tried to balance everything else on your plate.

These things happen, and they're normal. You should never feel bad about getting off track. It happens to everyone at some point in time. What is important, however, is that you recognize *why* you got off track so that you can prevent it in the future. If you know that the last time you tried to exercise regularly a busy schedule forced you to get off track, you can plan this time to figure out ways to fit in small amounts of walking throughout the day, no matter how busy it is. Or if you felt that you couldn't stay on track before due to a lack of support, you can work to find ways to increase your support, such as enlisting an exercise buddy or joining a walking group instead of trying to do it all on your own.

## Staying motivated with your walking routine

In order to increase your motivation and keep it high, you first have to understand what causes your motivation to decrease in the first place. Once you've discovered your biggest motivation suckers, you can start to strategize ways to overcome them. Take one of the biggest reasons motivation decreases: boredom. Boredom usually occurs when your workout never varies. If you do the exact same thing day after day, not only do you become mentally bored, but your results can stagnate as well, further decreasing motivation.

To beat boredom, think of all the simple ways you can add variety to your walking workout. For example, you can

- **Change your scenery.** If you walk outdoors, try walking a new route to mix things up. If you typically walk indoors, try venturing outdoors a few times per week or switch the location of your indoor walk. For instance, instead of walking on a treadmill, go mall walking one day for a different atmosphere and some interesting people-watching. You can even find interesting routes and make a movie of your walk(s) with GoPro, which is a wearable video camera, and share it with your friends on social media.

- **Challenge yourself.** Aim to increase your speed, your distance, or the intensity of your walk. Your walk can feel more exciting when you change it up and challenge yourself. You can even set goals for yourself, such as working to shave a minute off the time it takes you to walk a mile over the course of a few weeks. Little challenges such as these can give you a fresh perspective on your workout.

- **Enlist a buddy.** There's no better way to increase support and add the "fun factor" to a workout than to share it with friends or family. Talk with those around you and see who is also interested in increasing their fitness level and improving health. Perhaps your spouse would love the opportunity to walk with you in the evenings. Or maybe a coworker has also been wanting to start walking on lunch breaks. Having someone walk with you, and knowing that person relies on you to walk with her, increases your accountability and makes you more likely to stick with your walking plan. In addition, having company makes your workout more enjoyable, so you look forward to it each day. Even communities in fitness apps can help motivate you.

✔ **Add equipment to make your workout more fun.** If your standard walk feels like it's becoming monotonous, focus on switching it up a bit. There's so much equipment on the market for walking, you may be surprised at what you find. You can use a walking stick to improve balance and add intensity to your workout. Or perhaps using resistance bands during your walk to increase strength and muscle mass may appeal to you. Even using a fitness gadget, such as a pedometer or another tracking tool, can be a great way to get more feedback on your fitness as well as improve motivation and the "fun factor" of your walk.

✔ **Focus on more than just weight-loss results.** When your only focus as you start to walk on a regular basis is the number on the scale, it's easy to feel unmotivated if that number fails to move one week. However, you can gain many benefits from walking that aren't just about your body weight. Your energy level may improve, and your stress levels may decrease. You may sleep better at night or see improvements in health levels such as cholesterol and blood pressure. You may lose inches around your waistline, indicating a decrease in dangerous belly fat. The list goes on and on. Keep a journal each week of all the positive changes you notice from walking, both physical and mental. And when you feel discouraged or as though the scale isn't changing fast enough, look back at this list to help you focus on *all* the amazing results you're experiencing.

# Goal Setting for Successful Walking

When it comes to overcoming obstacles and staying on track with your walking plan, setting goals is critical to success. Now, you may be thinking, "I already have a goal — to lose weight!" And yes, that's true. That's your long-term, ultimate goal.

But if you focus only on the big, long-term goal, it's easy to start to feel discouraged and lose motivation. Say you set a goal to lose 50 pounds. This is certainly an achievable goal, but achieving it is going to take time. If every time you weigh yourself, all you focus on is losing a total of 50 pounds, you'll never feel excited when you see a drop of *just* one or two pounds. Instead, you'll think about how long it took to lose those few pounds and how much longer it will take to lose the rest. This type of thinking can be defeating and can decrease your motivation before you even get started.

However, if you instead focus on small goals that will ultimately lead to you achieving the long-term goal, you'll most likely feel much more accomplished and motivated. With the same long-term goal of losing 50 pounds, if you instead focus on a smaller goal of losing 10 pounds, you'll achieve your goal much faster. Every time you achieve your 10-pound goal, you can focus on the next goal of losing an additional 10 pounds. By doing this, your sense of achievement increases, you build more confidence in yourself, and before you know it, you achieve your long-term goal. You can write goals in a journal, or use a website or app to access charts and easy tools that give you access to your progress anywhere, anytime.

It's also important to set more than just one goal for yourself when it comes to walking for weight loss. Sure, your main goal most likely is to achieve your long-term weight-loss goal, but what about other goals that aren't so weight focused? The thing is, you can't entirely control the scale. You can control what you eat and how active you are, but the number on the scale can fluctuate due to reasons beyond your control. Perhaps you're holding onto water weight due to a medication you have to be on. Or maybe a hormone shift is impacting the number on the scale. These things won't last forever, and they won't cause real weight gain, but fluid shifts can certainly make the number on the scale less exciting. If your only focus is on this number, it can be hard to stay motivated when you don't see the scale changing as fast as you'd hoped.

Having additional goals to focus on, such as improvements in how you feel, your health, or a change in measurements, can increase your motivation and let you see how your walking routine is really impacting your body and overall health. Having at least three or four goals to focus on is key to staying motivated for long-term success.

## Setting goals for your health

Achieving an appropriate body weight is, of course, important for your health; however, even before reaching your ultimate weight-loss goal, you may start to see marked improvements in your overall health. Making sure that you notice these improvements can help you stay motivated, even if your weight-loss progress slows or stalls at times.

Before starting a walking routine, it's helpful to get a baseline of some basic health measurements. Then, you can compare this baseline to your new measurements periodically to assess the changes and improvements in your overall health. Some measurements you may want to track include the following:

✔ Blood pressure levels

✔ Blood lipids, including total cholesterol, LDL-cholesterol, HDL-cholesterol, and triglyceride levels

✔ Blood glucose levels

✔ Hemoglobin A1c (a 3-month average of blood glucose levels) if you've been diagnosed with diabetes or prediabetes

✔ Bone density if you've been diagnosed with osteopenia or osteoporosis

✔ Inflammatory markers such as C-reactive protein and homocysteine levels if you have (or are at an increased risk of having) heart disease

Speak with your healthcare provider about what health markers impact you the most and know your numbers. Once you know your baseline, you can track any changes and improvements over time to keep yourself motivated beyond just the number on the scale. See my website for labs and other tests that may be useful, especially if you have no or high-cost health insurance. Many tests are quite reasonably priced.

## Setting goals for weight loss

When setting weight-loss goals, it's important to be realistic. If you set a weight-loss goal that's too ambitious, it may be impossible to achieve. You're only setting yourself up for disappointment and failure. Instead, start by setting a realistic, achievable weight goal. You can always adjust your goal over time, but don't make it too lofty to start. You also want to make sure it's a healthy goal. For instance, if you're a 5-foot, 8-inch female, a goal of weighing 110 pounds is neither healthy nor realistic. Achieving that goal would mean being underweight, which brings with it its own set of health concerns.

As you are losing weight, don't forget to focus on measurements in addition to the scale. The number on the scale can fluctuate for many reasons, but your waist circumference doesn't fluctuate nearly as much. Measuring your waist circumference at the start of your walking plan and remeasuring every few weeks can help you assess how much unhealthy visceral (or belly) fat you are losing. Chapter 1 outlines how to take this measurement as well as the goal ranges for this number.

No matter how dedicated you are, you shouldn't expect to lose 5 pounds per week. Sure, during the first week of a weight-loss plan you may see a rapid decrease as you lose water weight as well as fat mass. But after that water weight is gone, you want to continue to lose mostly fat mass. Losing more than 2 pounds per week means you aren't just losing fat, but muscle as well. Because muscle is what makes up the majority of your metabolism, you want to maintain as much of it as possible. A healthy weight-loss progression is to lose weight between ½ and 2 pounds per week. Losing any amount within that range is making great progress!

It's important to remember that when it comes to weight loss, it's the averages over time that matter. One week you may see a weight loss, one week you may see no change, and another you may even see a small gain. However, if you take the average rate of weight loss over the period of a few weeks, that will show you your actual progress. If your progress averages out to ½ to 2 pounds per week, you're doing great. If it slows to less than this, you may want to assess whether you've already achieved a healthy weight. If not, it may be time to adjust your walking workout to speed up your results.

# Walking after an Injury

An untimely injury can sideline your walking and prevent you from achieving your goals. Repeated injury or an improperly treated injury can lead to chronic pain and frustration, which can also impact your motivation to continue to walk on a regular basis. Before starting a walking routine, it's critical to meet with your physician and discuss your planned exercise program. Discuss the most common injuries and those that pose the greatest risk for you. Your healthcare provider can help you determine your individual risk factors as well as the most effective precautions you can take to avoid injury.

Chapter 6 provides a detailed listing of the most common walking-related injuries and the signs and symptoms of each. If you start to notice pain, don't ignore it.

Treating an injury before it becomes worse is key to getting back to walking more quickly. Ignoring an injury can lead to chronic pain or significantly increase recovery time, taking you out of your exercise routine for longer than you may have planned.

Injuries can be major obstacles when it comes to staying on track with your walking routine, so learning the most common causes of injury and avoiding them can decrease your risk of developing one. Some of the main reasons injuries develop during walking are due to the following:

- ✔ Improper walking technique.

- ✔ Improper or unsupportive footwear.

- ✔ Repeated walking on very hard surfaces or uneven terrain.

- ✔ Failing to warm up, cool down, or stretch.

- ✔ Doing too much too soon. Slowly increasing the intensity, speed, and duration of your walking workout is key to decreasing injury risk.

Many of the most common walking injuries are preventable if you take steps to decrease your risk. Walking is a fantastic, low-impact form of exercise, but just like any form of movement, if not done correctly, it can lead to injury. Make sure your walking technique is correct (see Chapter 6), you warm up and cool down properly, and you always wear supportive footwear (see Chapter 5) when walking. The less risk of injury, the less your risk of being sidelined or losing motivation.

# Chapter 18

# Maintaining Your Weight Loss

. . . . . . . . . . . . . . . . . . . . . . . . . . . . . . . . . . . . . . . . . . . . . . . . . . . . . .

## In This Chapter

▶ Understanding the concepts of weight and health maintenance

▶ Determining the best ways to keep pounds off

▶ Coping with the most common obstacles to weight maintenance

▶ Adapting your walking routine to maintain your new weight

. . . . . . . . . . . . . . . . . . . . . . . . . . . . . . . . . . . . . . . . . . . . . . . . . . . . . .

*I*f you've now reached your weight loss and measurement goals, you may be wondering what's next. Walking off the weight isn't just something you do to quickly shed pounds only to go back to old behaviors and regain the weight. Getting active and staying active is a lifestyle change. And if you stick with this lifestyle change, you can maintain your results. Making lifestyle changes is how you not only lose weight, but keep it off for good. And that's the whole point of a weight-loss plan. You want to make sure that what you do to lose weight is something you can continue to stick with so that you can stay at your goal weight for years to come and continue to not only look great, but feel great and stay healthy as well.

Unlike some weight-loss plans that show you how to achieve your goals but fail to show you how to maintain them, I don't leave you hanging. This chapter provides you with clear-cut guidelines and tips on how to maintain the weight you have lost for good. After reading this chapter, you'll be able to determine when you have reached your goal weight and exactly what you need to do to stay at this weight once and for all.

## What Is Weight Maintenance?

Have you ever wondered what weight maintenance really is? It's basically just maintaining a consistent body weight over a period of months and years. Instead of reaching a goal weight only to start to regain weight, creating that yo-yo effect, weight maintenance means achieving a healthy body weight for you, one you can maintain for a very long period of time, without feeling the need to starve yourself.

Now, keep in mind that no one is the exact same weight every day. Weight can fluctuate on the scale for many reasons. So, when it comes to weight maintenance, I recommend aiming to stay within a weight range rather than at one specific weight. I suggest using a 3- to 5-pound weight range. So for instance, if your long-term goal is 135 pounds, your weight may fluctuate between 133–137 pounds. However, if your weight begins to slowly creep above this range, you can immediately increase the duration or intensity of your walking workout, make adjustments to your meal plan, and keep records of your food and exercise to help you stay within your goal range.

## Determining your weight-loss goals

What were the goals you set for yourself when you first picked up this book and decided you wanted to lose weight and improve your health? Did they include reaching a specific goal weight or BMI? Did you want to reach a certain pant size or attain a certain health goal, such as a normal blood pressure reading or glucose level?

Typically, once you reach your long-term goal, you are ready to move into your maintenance plan. Not everyone moves into maintenance at the same time or for the same reason. You may have already met your goal of losing 5 inches around your waist but still not be ready to transition to maintenance. Or, perhaps you were at a healthy body weight to begin with, but needed to lower your blood sugar levels. Once those levels are normal and staying that way, then it's time to transition into maintenance. Consider the following questions to assess whether you're ready to transition to the maintenance plan:

- ✔ Are you at your goal weight?
- ✔ Is your BMI within the ideal range?
- ✔ Are your health goals, such as blood pressure, cholesterol, and blood sugar, within the normal range?
- ✔ Is your waist circumference within the ideal range?

## What is the healthiest weight for you?

If your rate of weight loss seems to have slowed or stopped, you may have hit a weight-loss plateau, or you may have reached a healthy body weight. If you have reached a plateau, changing the duration, frequency, or intensity of your walking plan can help. If, however, you've been on track with your meal plan and exercise routine, it's possible that you aren't at a plateau at all and instead have achieved a healthy weight for you. You can go online to my website at `www.erinpalinski-author.com` for a list of free BMI and fitness calculators to help you determine whether you are at the healthiest weight for you.

Although you may have set a different weight as your goal in your mind, it's important to make sure the weight you're aiming for is a healthy weight for your height and gender, not one that's too low or unrealistic to maintain. If you set an unrealistic goal, you may feel like you've stalled before reaching this goal, when in reality, you've actually achieved a healthy weight.

Also, body weight is not the sole indicator of whether you have reached your goals. If your progress has stalled but your waist circumference and other health measurements (such as blood pressure and blood sugar) are all within the normal range, it's quite possible that you are at your goal and should now focus on maintenance.

When setting a weight-loss goal for yourself, there are many factors you should consider. Are you very athletic with a large amount of muscle mass? Do you have a large bone structure? (This is usually evident by a large wrist circumference.) If so, you may be on the higher end of the healthy weight scale, as muscle and bone mass weigh more on a scale than fat mass.

## Using measurements to determine whether you have met your goals

Your waist circumference is an indication of the amount of *visceral fat,* or belly fat, you have. The more belly fat you have, the greater your risk of future health complications such as type 2 diabetes and heart disease. Because walking is one of the best ways to shrink this dangerous fat, watching for changes in waist circumference can be a way to determine when you have achieved a healthy body weight.

Although the number on the scale may not reach the ideal number you had in your head, if your waist circumference falls within a healthy body range, you can be assured that the weight and inches you have lost have already made a big impact on your overall health.

To help reduce your risk of medical complications, waist circumference should be as follows:

✔ Less than 35 inches for women

✔ Less than 40 inches for men

> ✔ Less than 31 inches for women of Asian decent
>
> ✔ Less than 35 inches for men of Asian decent

Achieving a waist circumference within the ideal range may also be an indication that you have achieved, or are close to achieving, your ideal weight and health goals. In addition to waist circumference, some of the technology I mention in Chapter 2 along with personal body fat scales and hand devices can help you determine whether you have achieved your ideal weight and health goals. You can find many of these products at Amazon.com as well as other retailers and sporting goods stores. My website also includes a list of many of these items, where they can be purchased, and coupons (when available) as well.

# Focusing on Health Maintenance

Most people want to lose weight for a number of reasons. Of course, looking better or fitting into a smaller clothing size may be a top priority. However, the improvements in health from reducing body weight should really be the main focus of any weight-loss plan. Although you may not see these changes as quickly as you see numbers decreasing on the scale, health improvements are very real and are incredibly beneficial to overall longevity and quality of life.

Having your health measurements such as cholesterol, blood pressure, and blood sugar (glucose) within the normal range can also be an indication that you have achieved your ideal weight range and are ready to shift from continued weight loss to weight maintenance. These measurements can help to assess your risk of diseases such as heart disease, metabolic syndrome, and diabetes. The closer you can get these numbers to a healthy range — and keep them there — the better off you will be in the long term.

A quick online search can help you find resources to determine healthy measurements for cholesterol, blood pressure, and blood sugar. Talk with your doctor about getting these important health factors checked.

Tables 18-1 to 18-3 show the ideal ranges for various health measurements to help you gauge whether you may have met your health and weight goals.

| Table 18-1 | Ideal Measurements for Cholesterol | |
|---|---|---|
| *Blood Lipids* | *Range* | *Risk Category* |
| **Total Cholesterol** | <170 mg/dL | Ideal |
| | <200 mg/dL | Desirable |
| **LDL-Cholesterol** | <100 mg/dL | Ideal |
| | 100–129 mg/dL | Desirable |
| **HDL-Cholesterol** | >60 mg/dL (men and women) | Ideal |
| | 40–59 mg/dL (men) | Desirable |
| | 50–59 mg/dL (women) | Desirable |
| **Triglycerides** | <150 mg/dL | Desirable |

| Table 18-2 | Ideal Measurements for Blood Pressure | |
|---|---|---|
| *Category* | *Systolic* | *Diastolic* |
| Normal | <120 mmHg | <80 mmHg |
| High | >130 mmHg | >90 mmHg |

| Table 18-3 | Ideal Measurements for Blood Sugar (Glucose) |
|---|---|
| *Glucose Levels (Fasting)* | *Category* |
| Normal | 70–99 mg/dL |
| Prediabetic | 100–125 md/dL |
| Diabetic | 126 mg/dL and greater |

# Congratulations! You've Reached Your Goal! Now What?

First, let me congratulate you on the fantastic progress you've made! It's a terrific accomplishment to reach your goal weight, and you should be so proud of yourself! All your hard work and dedication have finally paid off. And, because of your efforts, your body not only looks better, but is so much healthier on the inside too!

Now that you're at your goal weight, you need to switch gears. Instead of focusing on weight loss, it's now time to focus on maintaining your current body weight. This is where a lot of people get a bit thrown off. You may be asking questions such as: Can I stop exercising? How much less can I walk? How much more food can I eat? Should I eat the same things I did as I lost the weight? If I change my meal plan or exercise routine, will the pounds pile back on?

## Factors that impact weight maintenance

The key to weight maintenance is moderation. You need to splurge on occasion or take a day off here and there from exercise, when needed, because maintaining weight is a lifelong journey. You can't expect yourself to be physically active all the time and eat perfectly every day.

It's also important to continue to implement the healthy behaviors that have helped you to reach your goal weight. Going back to old habits will just cause the weight to come back on. Instead, you want to slightly adjust your exercise routine (and your meal plan if you made dietary changes), but continue to keep an eye on the scale. I don't want you to get carried away with weighing yourself, but you should step on the scale at least once every week. This way, if your weight begins to creep up slightly, you can automatically make a few small changes in your food intake and exercise level to get that extra pound or two off before it becomes 10 or 20 pounds that you need to lose.

## How tracking plays a role in long-term success

Weight maintenance is a bit of trial and error. You can slowly change your walking plan or increase your food intake, but to know exactly how much extra you can eat or what intensity and duration of exercise work best for you, you need to keep track of what you eat and your exercise routine in addition to your weight for a few weeks. The extent to which you can adjust your exercise routine or meal plan depends on your age, activity level, gender, height, and whether your weight-loss progress slowed on its own or you consistently lost weight until you decided you no longer needed to lose anymore.

Tracking is very important when it comes to successful weight maintenance. If you fail to track, you may not be aware when weight begins to creep back on, or worse yet, you may not be sure why weight is coming back on. As you work toward tracking your behaviors, make sure to keep a record of the following:

- ✔ **The details of your walking workouts:** Include the distance you walk and the length of your walks, as well as the speed, incline, resistance, and any other factors that impact the intensity of your walking routine. Also track how many days per week you exercise.

- ✔ **Your food intake:** Include everything you eat and drink, the amounts of each, any additional condiments or additional sources of calories (for example, cream and sugar in coffee), and the timing of your meals and snacks.

- ✔ **Your weight:** Weigh in around once per week so you notice right away if your weight is beginning to creep back up on the scale.

- ✔ **Your measurements:** Take your measurements about once a month. Keep an eye out for any changes in waist circumference, which may indicate an increase in visceral fat.

## *Altering your walking plan to maintain your weight*

In addition to keeping an eye on your portions, it's very important to stay active. In fact, regular exercise is more important during maintenance than ever before — even more important than when you were trying to lose weight. Research has shown the majority of people who have lost a significant amount of weight and have kept it off long term perform some form of physical activity or structured exercise on a regular basis.

Maintaining your weight is a lifelong process, which means you have to be active for life. And if you do the exact same exercise day in and day out, for years and years, you may very well get bored with it. But exercise doesn't have to be boring; in fact, it should never be boring. It should be fun! That's what helps you stick with it! That's what makes walking such a great choice for not only losing weight, but keeping it off as well. It's so versatile.

You can walk anywhere, anytime. Once you have reached your goal weight, you may choose to go for a hike one day, take a stroll around your neighborhood the next, or just aim to reach at least 10,000 steps another day. Any of these strategies keeps you moving, helping to keep weight off as well as keep your body healthy.

But don't forget: It's important to challenge yourself every once in a while too. Even if you are walking for fun and mixing your walk up once in a while to prevent boredom, it's still easy to fall into a rut if you're doing the same thing over and over. So think of a way to push yourself a bit so you are always striving to get stronger and faster. For instance, sign up for a 5K or 10K race and work on improving your walking speed or distance times. If you have always walked at a casual pace, try mixing up your walking plan with a brisk walk or change the terrain to add in a bit of incline. If you have always power walked, switch it up at times with a slow-paced, stress-relieving walk.

Varying when and where you walk can help prevent boredom as well. If you always walk indoors on a treadmill, try taking your walking workout outdoors and enjoying a change of scenery. If you want to stay indoors, mix up where you walk: Take a stroll at a shopping center one day versus always working out at the gym. The more you challenge yourself and mix up your workout, the more fit you will become and the easier it will be to stay motivated to stick with your activity of choice.

## Altering your meal plan to maintain weight loss

When it comes to maintaining your weight loss, diet plays just as important a role as staying active. If you continue to walk daily but start to consume more calories than you once did, you'll see weight begin to climb back on. If you were following a structured meal plan to promote weight loss while walking, you can typically be a bit more flexible with your food intake after you have reached your goal. Most people can maintain their weight while adding back between 100 and 500 calories per day from a weight-loss meal plan. The amount depends on your age, activity level, gender, height, and whether your weight-loss progress slowed on its own or you consistently lost weight until you decided you no longer needed to lose anymore.

If you are more than 40 years old, perform less than 30 minutes of moderate-paced walking per day, are female, are of short stature, or hit a weight-loss plateau at a desirable body weight, then generally you'll want to add back about 100 to 300 calories per day for weight maintenance. If you are less than 40 years old, a male, tall in stature, or very active, or if your weight-loss progress never slowed or stalled, you may be able to add back in up to 500 calories per day to maintain your weight loss.

Keep in mind that weight maintenance can be very individualized. If you are consistent with both your walking plan and meal plan, and you find that after two to three weeks you are still losing weight, add an additional 100 calories per day for one week and monitor your weight. Repeat this until you maintain your weight for at least two weeks in a row. The opposite applies as well: If you are following a consistent plan and your weight is slightly creeping upward, cut back by 100 calories per day for a week and re-assess your progress.

To put it in perspective, 100 calories is generally equal to any of the following:

✔ 1 slice of bread or ½ cup of cereal

✔ 1 baseball-sized piece of fruit

✔ 1 cup of lowfat milk

✔ 3 ounces of lean protein

✔ 2 teaspoons of olive oil

Meal planning, portion control, and tracking are essential when it comes to monitoring your calorie and food intake to maintain your weight loss.

If you find your schedule and lifestyle are too hectic to plan meals in advance, or if you struggle to find the time to cook for yourself on a regular basis, many companies now offer home delivery service of healthy, calorie-controlled meals. These services can range from as low as $10 per day and up depending on your location, food selection, and calorie needs. A listing of companies that offer meal delivery services is available on my website.

# Overcoming Weight Maintenance Obstacles

One of the biggest obstacles that most individuals face when trying to prevent weight regain is sticking with the changes they made to lose weight in the first place. As you work toward increasing the amount of walking you do each day to help shed pounds and inches, it's important to remember that moving more isn't just a quick fix. It's vital for overall health and wellness as well as weight management. For that reason, being active on a regular basis needs to become part of your daily routine more than anything.

In this section, I give you some tips for making your lifestyle changes — and your new ideal weight — permanent.

## Lifestyle changes that keep off the pounds

In order to make physical activity a daily habit, you can focus on it in a number of ways. You can look at increasing your overall physical activity, or daily movement, just by making sure to wear a pedometer each day to track and record your daily steps. You can incorporate regular walks into your day as part of a routine you follow with your family, coworkers, or friends.

You can also focus social gatherings and events on physical activity, such as taking a walk while talking and catching up, rather than food. The more you make movement part of your overall daily routine, the easier it will be to keep the pounds off long term.

Eating a well-balanced diet and monitoring your portions are also key to preventing weight regain. There's no point in making drastic changes you can't live with, because you'll fall right back into your old habits. The best strategy is to make gradual changes that you can continue to follow long term to improve your health and maintain a healthy body weight. To do this, try to incorporate most, if not all, of the following dietary principles into your regular meal plan for a healthier, slimmer you:

- ✔ **Eating is important.** Don't skip meals or you will become too hungry, eat too fast, and ultimately eat too much.

- ✔ **Transition to whole grains.** These grains are richer in nutrients and fiber, keeping you full longer and preventing nasty spikes in insulin, which trigger belly fat storage.

- ✔ **Eat more produce.** Vegetables and fruits are key to good nutrition. They're loaded with filling fiber, have few calories, and are packed full of disease-fighting antioxidants.

- ✔ **Avoid inflammatory foods.** Inflammation triggers belly fat storage and is an underlying factor in many disease states. Avoid refined carbohydrates, foods rich in saturated fats and trans fats, and highly processed foods.

- ✔ **Eat at least one good source of healthy fat every day.** Monounsaturated fats and omega-3 fatty acids help to fight both belly fat and inflammation. These fats are essential to maintaining a desirable body weight as well as preventing disease.

- ✔ **Drink at least 8 to 10 cups of water every day.** Hydration keeps your energy level up, fills you up to help you reduce your portions at meals and snacks, and helps your metabolism function at its peak. So drink up!

- ✔ **Practice mindful eating.** This is a very important principle! You need to recognize your body's hunger and satiety cues to be able to maintain a healthy body weight for life.

## Making lifestyle changes that stick

One main way to keep off the weight you have lost is to realize that you can't be perfect. No one is perfect — especially when it comes to exercise or food. And, if you try to be perfect 100 percent of the time with your walking routine or what you are eating, you're going to burn yourself out.

### Splurge once in a while

Part of weight maintenance is understanding that you'll be more active some days than others and that all foods have a place in your diet — some just more often than others. If you're a junk food junky, you can't expect to never have a chip for the rest of your life. That's completely unrealistic. Yes, you can expect to not eat chips every day (that wouldn't be good for your waistline or health), but an occasional splurge is fine. It's actually healthy. Think about it like this: Imagine you are back in school studying for a huge exam. If you study every waking hour, you start to forget what you were studying for in the first place and may actually do worse on the exam, right? The same holds true with healthy eating and exercise. If you obsess over your food choices and scrutinize every morsel that enters your mouth, you'll eventually get so sick of doing this that you'll say "the heck with this" and shove whatever you feel like in your mouth.

And the same goes for walking. If you're inactive for a few days and then decide to walk 6 miles to make up for it one day, not only will you burn out, but you could also injure yourself, sidelining yourself from exercise for a long period of time. And that can put you right back where you started.

### Follow the 80/20 rule

Health is all about balance. And that's why I want you to follow my 80/20 rule when you're working to maintain your goal weight. I want you to focus 80 percent of the time on making healthy lifestyle changes, such as walking on a regular basis for at least 30 minutes most days and eating a well-balanced diet. Then 20 percent of the time, you have room to veer off track a bit. This is your "splurge." You may choose to have one day a week where you take a rest day and be slightly less active or have a "splurge" meal. Or maybe you prefer to have a small snack twice a week where you don't exactly make the healthiest choice. These little breaks here and there are good for you. They prevent you from experiencing burnout or feeling deprived. If you start to feel deprived or burned out, you tend to go back to the old behaviors that lead to weight gain in the first place.

Making lifestyle changes you can stick with is really vital to your weight-loss success. In fact, it's really the *only* way to keep weight off for good. That's why I keep saying it, because it's so essential if you want to be successful long term. It's also important to be realistic with the lifestyle changes you make. You need to make sure the changes you do make to your eating and exercise habits are really things you can see yourself doing long term.

### Make small changes

There are many small changes you can make that lead to very big results. And any change you make, no matter how small — assuming it's a change you can stick with — is terrific. Here are some of the small changes I find most effective in promoting big results for long-term success:

- ✔ **Manage stress.** Figure out what stresses you and find a way to manage it (without food!). Stress can really pile on belly fat due to the increased production of stress hormones. It can also increase blood pressure and insulin resistance. Unfortunately, you can't avoid stress, but you can pay attention to find out what the biggest stressors are in your life. Once you recognize them, see whether there are changes you can make to reduce these stressors. Even tiny changes that reduce stress slightly have a large impact on your health and belly fat! And remember, one of the best ways to fight stress is with exercise, so get walking!

- ✔ **Be prepared!** When you fail to plan, you plan to fail — I'm sure you've heard that many times. But it's true, especially for weight-loss success. Keeping weight off is work. It involves planning ahead to make sure you have the time to walk. Know exactly when, where, and how long you will walk to make sure it actually happens. Have the right food on hand to prevent you from becoming too hungry or making poor food choices.

- ✔ **Plan your meals in advance.** In addition to cooking in advance, planning what you will eat throughout the week is not only a great way to ensure you have the food you need on hand, but it also cuts down on those "what should I eat" moments. And, planning out menus in advance is a great way to reduce your grocery bill!

- ✔ **Track your activity.** Whether or not you are walking for a set length of time each day, tracking your steps to gauge your total daily steps can be very eye-opening. If you typically walk 10,000 steps per day and one week your average drops to less than 4,000 steps per day, you may be on the path toward regaining weight. If that happens, you can identify it right away and get moving to prevent weight regain.

# Weight Maintenance Walking Routine

When it comes to walking to keep the weight off, there's no set plan that works for everyone. Keeping the weight off requires an individual plan based on how you walked to lose the weight. If you focused on just increasing your overall daily steps to lose weight, then you need to make only small adjustments to continue to keep the weight off. Look at the total number of steps you walk, on average, every day.

For general health, you want to aim to walk a minimum of 10,000 steps every day, although you can always aim to walk additional steps. If you walked 12,000 to 14,000 steps per day to lose weight, decreasing your total daily steps by about 2,000 to 4,000 steps after reaching your goal weight (without changing your meal plan) will usually result in weight maintenance rather than continued weight loss.

If you incorporated any of the fitness walking routines in this book to lose weight, you have options when it comes to maintaining your progress. You don't want to stop exercising entirely. That would be damaging to your health as well as your weight-loss progress. Instead, you can adjust the duration, frequency, or intensity of your walk on a regular basis:

- ✔ **Duration:** If you were walking for 60 minutes at once for most of your walking workouts, you can scale down some or all of your workouts to 30–45 minutes most days of the week.

- ✔ **Frequency:** If you were walking six days per week, you can choose to lower the frequency with which you walk to five days per week to maintain health benefits while keeping your weight steady.

- ✔ **Intensity:** If you were walking at a high intensity by increasing your speed or incline level, you can slightly reduce your speed (add one or two extra minutes per mile walked) or lower your incline level 2 or 3 percent to lower the intensity while keeping the duration of the workout, and your weight, the same.

When it comes to maintaining weight, no two people are exactly alike. Play around with adjusting your walking workout and see what works for you. Make sure to continue to weigh yourself regularly. If you go from walking 60 minutes per day to 30 minutes and notice a slight weight gain after a month, try walking 45 minutes per day instead to see whether that works better for you in regard to weight maintenance.

Staying on track with your walking routine also means making sure that it stays enjoyable. The more fun you have while walking, the more likely you are to stick with it. Depending on where you live and the time of year, you can incorporate hiking or even snowshoeing into your walking routine.

Walking tours can also be a fantastic way to change up your walking routine (or stick with it when traveling). A variety of walking tours are available, from sightseeing to ghost-hunting. You can even download audio walking tours to your iPhone before heading out. No matter where you are, you can find domestic and international audio and in-person walking tours. A full list can be found on my website at www.erinpalinski-author.com. You don't have to travel to have fun, either. You can create or join a local walking group, or take advantage of the time you spend walking to learn a new skill, such as a new language, by listening to audio files.

If you find your motivation is waning, get your friends and family involved in your walk. You can be cheered on by your loved ones or even have them donate to your favorite charity for every mile you walk with websites such as www.krowdfit.com. If you want to feel great about walking, look into some websites and apps, which I list on my website, that will even donate to a charity for every mile that your walk! It doesn't get much more motivating than that!

# Part V
# The Part of Tens

the part of tens

**web extras**

Enjoy an additional Part of Tens chapter online at
www.dummies.com/extras/walkingtheweightoff.

# In this part . . .

✔ Learn the best ways to maximize your weight-loss results with easy techniques to implement during your workout.

✔ Discover the most essential tools for a walker and how they can help you to achieve your results more quickly.

# Chapter 19

# Ten Ways to Maximize Your Walking Workout

After you've been following your walking workout on a regular basis, you may feel as though it's time to increase the intensity of your workout. Perhaps your weight loss has stalled, and you want to increase the number of calories you burn during each workout. Perhaps you no longer feel challenged during your walking workout, and you're ready to push yourself a bit harder.

Sticking with the same walking routine day after day can start to feel monotonous. Worse yet, if your body becomes too accustomed to your workout, you'll start to see fewer results. Changing your workout can not only help you to challenge yourself further, but it can also prevent boredom and keep you energized and excited to get walking and stay walking.

No matter what the reason, you can use any of these ten ways, or a combination of them, to maximize your workout and your results.

As always, make sure to consult your physician before starting or changing any exercise routine.

## Head for the Hills

Walking uphill is one of the easiest ways to add an incline to your walk. By walking on an incline, you can significantly increase the calorie expenditure of every minute of your walking workout. The higher the incline, the more you challenge the muscles in your core and lower body. Therefore, the higher the incline and the more often you walk on an incline, the faster you'll see results. Not only will incline walking help to speed weight loss, but it will also help to tone and tighten your glutes and core.

To get started, examine your outdoor walking routine. Look for terrain that has a slight incline and see whether you can add this into your typical route. Start with a mild incline and, over time, challenge yourself to steeper and steeper hills. If you want to really get technical when it comes to your incline, you can even use a clinometer to measure the steepness of your hills by downloading a free clinometers app on your iPhone or Android. If your walking routine is snowshoeing, you'll need FitClimb (www.fitclimb.com).

Keep in mind that if you suffer from back or knee issues, walking at an incline may not be appropriate for you. Always follow the advice of your physician.

# Race Yourself

No matter how fast or slow your current walking pace, you can always work on slowly increasing your individual walking speed. The faster your walking speed, the more calories per minute you burn. And the more calories you burn, the quicker you can lose weight and keep it off. If you're not sure how to get started with increasing your speed, try this: Walk at your normal pace and time yourself to see how long it takes you to walk 1 mile. No matter how long it takes, the next time you go for a walk, try to walk slightly faster and see whether you can complete the mile 30 seconds faster.

Once you have accomplished this, aim to shave another 30 seconds off your mileage time. Repeat this over and over again until you can successfully walk a mile in 15 minutes or less. If you are tracking your progress through a heart rate monitor, GPS, or fitness app, you can use Strava to track all your activity. Upload your activities from your GPS Garmin, Android, or iPhone, and Strava will automatically log all your workouts, and allow you to compare and compete with yourself or other walkers on leaderboards. I list devices that are compatible with Strava on my website at www.erinpalinski-author.com.

# Step It Up

It may sound simple, but adding a few bouts of stair climbing to your walk can make your workout significantly more challenging. Walking up stairs challenges all the muscles in your lower body and core. Challenging these muscles helps you to increase strength and muscle mass, boosting metabolism. In addition, as these muscles strengthen, they help to tone and tighten your lower body, speeding your loss of inches. Stair climbing can also increase bone density in your hips and spine, helping to fight against osteoporosis.

# Pump Iron

Adding resistance training, such as using dumbbells to perform strength-training exercises either during your walking workout or directly before or after can speed results in a variety of ways. First, strength-training exercises help to build and strengthen muscle.

The more muscle mass you have, the higher your metabolism, which causes you to burn more calories throughout the day. In addition, strengthening muscle helps to tone and tighten areas of the body such as the thighs and core, helping you to lose inches. And finally, adding resistance training increases the intensity of your workout, meaning that you burn more calories during the duration of your workout, maximizing your weight-loss efforts.

To get started, view the exercises in the Resistance Walking and Total Body Workout Walking plans in Chapter 10. Incorporating these exercises at least two times per week can help you to see results quickly, and most importantly, maintain your results long term.

If using dumbbells for upper-body strengthening isn't appealing, you can try using walking poles that keep your arms moving. Health Mark, Inc. makes walking poles that even have a built-in pedometer, such as the Alumilite Trekking Pole. You can find them and others on wayfair.com. You can also use walking weights with hand straps, such as Gold's Gym Soft Walking Weights; start light and work up to heavier weight as your muscles strengthen.

# Mix It Up

Not only can performing the same exercise day in and day out become boring (which can make it challenging to continue with your exercise routine), but your body also can become accustomed to your workout plan. When this happens, your body is no longer as challenged as it once was. And when your body no longer has to work as hard to complete an exercise, you end up burning fewer calories during your workout.

To prevent this from happening, it's important to mix up your walking routine. You don't want to walk in the same exact way day after day, or your results will start to stagnate. The walking programs provided in this book incorporate variety to maximize results. However, even if you don't follow these programs, you can mix up your workout on your own to see faster results. From day to day, vary your speed, the length of your walk, the incline level, and even where you walk. For instance, one day walk outside on a flat surface for 45 minutes. The next day, walk inside on a treadmill for 30 minutes, but at a faster speed. The following day, walk for 45 minutes incorporating an elevation in incline every ten minutes. The more you vary your workout, the better and faster your results!

## Add Intervals

Interval training can sound complicated, but it really isn't. The practice is just one of varying the intensity of your workout throughout the duration of the entire workout. When it comes to walking, this can be done by varying your speed or your incline. For example, to vary your speed, if you choose to walk for 30 minutes, you can incorporate intervals by walking at a moderate pace for 5 minutes, followed by walking as fast as you can for 1 minute, and then returning back to the moderate pace and repeating this pattern for the duration of the walk.

Intervals can also be added with incline. For instance, you can walk on a flat surface for five minutes, then walk at a high incline or up stairs for one minute, and then return back to the flat surface for an additional five minutes and repeat. This practice can be a great way to not only boost your results, but to keep your workout exciting as well.

## Focus on Daily Activity and Structured Walks

If you've been performing a structured walk at least a few times per week for exercise and aren't seeing the results you expected, then you also want to focus on your level of daily activity. Research has shown that sometimes when individuals start an exercise program, they actually become less active the rest of the day. So now, even though you burn additional calories during your walking workout, being less active the rest of the day causes your metabolism to be slower, leading to slow or stalled weight-loss results.

To prevent this, don't just focus on a fitness walk each day; make sure to also track your overall daily movement. This tracking can easily be done by wearing a pedometer for the duration of the day or a fitness tracker that even tracks sleep patterns. Put a pedometer on as soon as you wake up in the morning and wear it until you go to bed at night. Make sure that on days when you are walking for exercise, you continue to get just as many steps (and hopefully more) than on days when you don't exercise. If you notice the number of steps you take throughout the day is low, work on picking it up by squeezing in short bouts of walking anywhere you can. Park farther away, walk the long way to the bathroom, or take two trips instead of one to put laundry away. The more you move, and the more often, the faster you will see results.

# Make It Last

If you feel as though your weight-loss results have slowed or stalled, try increasing the time during which you walk each day. Even as little as five extra minutes of walking each day of the week can result in increased weight loss and improved health. If you walk for a set period of time each day, slowly add one to two minutes to this time each day. Aim to add anywhere from 5 to 30 minutes to your current walk. The longer you walk, the quicker you'll see results.

# Incorporate Technology

There are so many gadgets and gizmos on the market today, from Fitbit integrated with digital scales to Garmin's vívosmart fitness tracker to mobile phone GPS mapping apps to simple pedometers, it can feel a little over-whelming. However, many fitness gadgets can actually help you increase the effectiveness of your walk and see results more quickly. Some fitness tools can track the speed and duration of your walk, so you can use these to increase your walking intensity steadily over time. Other gadgets just make walking more fun, and the more you enjoy your workout, the more likely you are to stick with it.

See Chapter 20 for a listing of some great technology that can help to enhance your walking experience as well as your results or go to my website for information on the various technologies available, how they work, and what may be best for you.

# Get Stretchy

To many walkers, stretching can be an afterthought; however, stretching on a regular basis can actually help to speed your fitness results. When you stretch, you boost circulation, bringing oxygen and vital nutrients to your muscles. When this occurs, muscles can repair and strengthen more quickly, helping to prevent walking-related injuries that can sideline your workout. In addition, stretching can increase your overall range of motion. As this occurs, your gait may improve, which can allow you to walk at a quicker pace, further enhancing your results. Foam rollers, stretching bands, and exercise balls are very useful ways to help enhance flexibility as well. You can purchase them at many sporting good stores as well as online at retailers.

Most important, stretching after your muscles are warm feels good. You feel energized and ready to hit the road. The better you feel, the more likely you are to push yourself to walk quicker, farther, or at a higher incline. And the more you're able to safely push yourself, the more effective each walk becomes and the faster you ultimately see results.

# Chapter 20

# Ten Essential Tools for Any Walker

*W*hether you have yet to start your walking program or are already a seasoned walker, certain tools can enhance the effectiveness of your walk as well as make your life as a walker easier. For instance, having the proper footwear doesn't just help you feel better as you walk, but it can also lessen the wear and tear walking takes on your body, decreasing your risk of injury. But knowing what type is best for you as a walker is critical in order to reap the benefits.

Although you don't have to have any tools as a walker other than your feet and supportive footwear, adding tools to your walking workout can help in a few ways. Some tools, such as new ways to track your walking workout, can make your workout feel more fun and exciting. And when you're excited about walking, you're more apt to do it on a regular basis. Other tools can make walking in varying climates more comfortable or even safer. And tools like these can allow you to walk no matter what the weather brings, preventing you from having to sideline your exercise plans.

Safety is also critical when it comes to walking, and many tools on the market can make walking as safe as possible, especially if you walk outdoors. Tools that help drivers see you when you're walking and tools that illuminate your walking path can prevent accidents and injuries. Tracking and location tools can help you plan and change your walking path, prevent you from becoming lost, or make it possible for others find you if you become injured and need help.

Many of the tools listed in this chapter are just fun to have. Sure, you don't have to have them to walk for exercise, but having them can make the journey even more fun. And when you're enjoying yourself, you want to keep enjoying yourself — which keeps you walking day after day!

This chapter provides an overview of some tools worth considering.

# A Baseline

As you get started with your walking plan, you no doubt have certain goals in mind. Perhaps these are to improve your overall health or achieve a certain body weight. However, if you don't know or remember where you started, it can be hard to track your progress and realize your accomplishments over time. First, have a baseline of your overall general health by having blood tests done before starting your walking program. I outline the most commonly recommended tests in Chapter 2, such as knowing your cholesterol and blood glucose levels. In addition, tests such as bone density can be performed before you begin your exercise routine, so you can track changes over time.

Also, know your current Body Mass Index (BMI), waist circumference, and body weight. Chapter 2 outlines how to determine your waist circumference and BMI as well. Knowing these numbers will allow you to easily track changes over time, and help you to stay motivated as you work towards achieving your ultimate goals.

# Proper Footwear

The most important part of walking is the right pair of shoes! Having properly fitting footwear is essential in preventing walking-related injuries and discomfort. Based on your health needs, you may need more specialized footwear. For example, individuals with diabetes need to make sure their footwear protects against blisters or any potential irritants to prevent wounds and infections. Even individuals with orthopedic issues such as bunions can benefit from specialized footwear.

In Chapter 5, I outline the various criteria for finding the best shoe for you based on where and how often you walk, your health history, and even the type of walking you do. Always make sure that your footwear fits well and is comfortable. One brand known for comfort is the Ryka Radiant shoe, but many other options may be appropriate for you depending on your needs. For specialized footwear options, follow the recommendations of your podiatrist.

# Water Bottle

Staying hydrated is key to good health when it comes to exercise. The more you exercise, the more you sweat, which means the more water you need to drink to replace what you have lost. Dehydration — even slight dehydration — can drain your energy levels and even lower your metabolism.

To help you stay hydrated, invest in a good water bottle you can carry with you throughout the day. When choosing a water bottle, look for brands that are BPA free, lightweight, and portable. If you want to drink while you walk (for instance, if you walk in very warm weather or for long periods of time outdoors), you may want to consider using a hydration pack that you can wear as well.

# Logbook

Keeping a log of your walking workouts, your progress, and even any struggles you may be having is a great way to help yourself stay on track with your long-term goals and evaluate your efforts over time. People who keep journals tend to be much more likely to achieve their desired results, and the same is true when it comes to logging your fitness progress. You can keep a log the old-fashioned way, with a paper and pencil. However, many websites and apps also allow you to easily track your progress online if that's easier for you.

When choosing an app or a website, look for one that can automatically sync with any wearable fitness tracker you may be using or any Bluetooth enabled scale to make tracking as easy as possible. If you have a smartphone, look for websites that offer companion smartphone apps so you can enter data whenever its convenient for you. Hundreds of websites and apps offer these features, ranging from Spark People (an advertising-based, free website) to Strava ($69 per year), which integrates with various fitness devices like pedometers, heart rate monitors, and scales via Bluetooth. My favorite is Fitbit, which comes free with its fitness trackers. Technology changes quickly, so check www.erinpalinski-author.com to see the latest recommendations and a buying guide to help you pick the best website or app (or manual journal) that suits your needs.

# Fitness Tracker

Fitness trackers are great devices because they allow you to track how many steps you've taken, how far you've walked, and other data such as calories burned and sleep patterns. There are many wearable and other fitness tracking devices, from low tech to high tech. If you are interested in a simple, low-tech device, using a basic pedometer is a great way to track your total steps and the distance you walk each day.

Among the more popular and higher-tech tracking devices are wearable wristband fitness trackers, such as Fitbit. This wristband can be worn 24 hours a day and track the number of steps you take, the calories you burn, and even your sleep patterns. You can wear it no matter what you're doing, from showering to sleeping. Because devices such as this are worn all day and all night, they provide a more accurate way to track your total daily activity and calories burned, helping you to reach your weight-loss goals more quickly.

## Digital Scale

When you are working to lose weight, having an accurate scale on hand is essential. Without weighing yourself, it can be hard to know whether your weight is changing. If you're in the market for a scale, I recommend getting a digital one that contains Bluetooth technology. This feature allows the scale to effortlessly send your weight, body fat percentage, and BMI over a wireless connection to the smartphone app or website that you use to monitor your diet and fitness progress.

When choosing a Bluetooth-enabled scale, make sure to choose one that works with your favorite app or website. One option that's great for Fitbit users is the Aria digital scale, which seamlessly integrates with the fitness tracker. Using a scale on a regular basis (once a week) allows you to track and monitor your progress so you can stay motivated or make changes to your plan as needed to maximize your results.

## Safety Supplies

Taking your safety into account is key, especially if you plan to walk outdoors. If you walk near traffic, make sure you wear reflective clothing to alert vehicles to your presence. If you walk in the dark, carrying a flashlight or even wearing a headlamp is ideal for making sure your walking path is illuminated to protect against slips and falls. And whenever you walk, carry a cellphone with you so you can call for help in case of an emergency. If you have a medical condition, such as diabetes, consider wearing a medical alert bracelet as well so that if you do need help, medical responders will be aware of your condition.

## Walking Weights

If you are looking to maximize the intensity of your workout, adding resistance is a great option. Resistance allows you to not only burn more calories per minute as you walk, but also to build muscle mass. The more muscle mass you have, the higher your metabolism, which helps you to not only lose weight, but to keep it off as well.

When choosing weights to walk with, make sure you select weights that are light enough to carry for the duration of your walk without sacrificing form. One great option is Gold's Gym Soft Walking Weights, which are available on `www.wayfair.com`. Before adding weights to your walking workout, however, make sure to discuss with your physician whether resistance training, especially while walking, is appropriate for you.

# Social Motivation

Although you most likely started your walking workout with the best intentions, at times it can be difficult to stay motivated or keep at it. However, staying on track and being consistent with your walking efforts is key to both losing weight and keeping it off long term. It helps a lot to have motivation from friends, family, walking partners, or fitness groups!

One of the most inspiring tools now available is social motivation through an app or website. Online fitness communities consist of members who have similar goals and challenges. Communicating with these members can keep you inspired to get going and give you additional tips and advice to overcome challenges you may face along the way. You can find many of these fitness communities by searching online, and some wearable fitness trackers even offer them with their tracking website or app dashboard. If you're a Fitbit user, your device come with a free fitness-tracking dashboard and a large community from which to get motivation. Combining the support of the online community with support at home is a recipe for success!

# A Plan!

No matter how big or small your goals are, achieving them isn't possible without a plan of action. Stating that you'll start to walk for weight loss is great, but unless you lay out exactly how you plan to do it, it may not happen. Just the act of picking up this book and reading it is the first step in creating a plan to begin walking off those extra pounds. The next step is detailing when, where, how often, and for how long you'll walk. You can utilize the walking plans from this book or even develop your own. But, whatever you decide, sit down and write out your walking plan. Once you have it in hand, it's easy to stick with it and start seeing results!

# Index

### • D •

## • T •

## • U •

# About the Author

Erin Palinski-Wade, RD, LDN, CDE, is a nationally recognized nutrition and fitness expert, spokesperson, and speaker. She has contributed her expertise to national media outlets such as the *CBS Early Show, The Doctors, ABC News, CBS News,* and *NBC News* along with a variety of newspapers, magazines, and radio shows. She is the author of *Belly Fat Diet For Dummies, 2 Day Diabetes Diet,* and coauthor of *Flat Belly Cookbook For Dummies.*

Erin runs a private practice in northern New Jersey where she works with private clients and corporations in the areas of weight management, diabetes education, disease prevention, health promotion, and fitness. Her website, www.erinpalinski.com, offers monthly nutrition newsletters including tips and recipes. Erin also runs the blog www.MommyhoodBytes.com where she provides "bytes" of information on nutrition, fitness, and motherhood. She can be found on Twitter @DietExpertNJ and on Facebook at www.facebook.com/erinpalinski.

# Dedication

This book is dedicated to everyone who wants to get motivated and get moving to attain a healthy body weight, improve their overall well being, and achieve optimal health.

This book is also dedicated to my loving and supportive family and friends who, without your constant support and belief in me, this book would not have been possible.

# Author's Acknowledgments

Thank you to my incredibly supportive family who, without your patience and confidence in me, I would not have able to achieve what I have. Thank you to my husband for always being there for me and believing in me. Thank you to my son, Joseph, for being the greatest blessing I could ever hope for. Thank you to all of my family and friends for your constant encouragement, especially my parents. Without your help and support, I would never be able to manage my hectic work schedule and home life. I also thank all of the wonderful nutrition professionals who I have had the pleasure to work with for your guidance, advice, and support, especially my wonderful coworker Susan Gralla, who helps to make Vernon Nutrition Center what it is!

And special thanks to everyone that made this book possible including literary agent Margot Hutchison, acquisitions editor Tracy Boggier, project editor Tim Gallan, copy editor Christy Pingleton, art coordinator Alicia South, Kristen Rath Photography, and fitness models Patrick Wade and Alyson Stark. I can't tell you how much I have appreciated all of your support, patience, and knowledge.

## Publisher's Acknowledgments

**Acquisitions Editor:** Tracy Boggier

**Project Editor:** Tim Gallan

**Copy Editor:** Christine Pingleton

**Art Coordinator:** Alicia B. South

**Production Editor:** Selvakumaran Rajendiran

**Cover Image:** ©iStock.com/Juanmonino